Dr. Pestana's Surgery Notes

FOURTH EDITION

Top 180 Vignettes for the Surgical Wards

Carlos Pestana, MD, PhD

KAPLAN

This publication is designed to provide accurate information in regard to the subject matter covered as of its publication date, with the understanding that knowledge and best practice constantly evolve. The publisher is not engaged in rendering medical, legal, accounting, or other professional service. If medical or legal advice or other expert assistance is required, the services of a competent professional should be sought. This publication is not intended for use in clinical practice or the delivery of medical care. To the fullest extent of the law, neither the Publisher nor the Editors assume any liability for any injury and/or damage to persons or property arising out of or related to any use of the material contained in this book.

USMLE® is a joint program of the Federation of State Medical Boards of the United States and the National Board of Medical Examiners, neither of which sponsors or endorses this product.

Table of Contents

About the Author

Carlos Pestana, MD, PhD, is currently an emeritus professor of surgery at the University of Texas Medical School at San Antonio. A native of the Canary Islands, Spain, Dr. Pestana graduated from medical school in Mexico City, ranking #1 in his class, and subsequently received a doctorate in surgery from the University of Minnesota, in conjunction with a 5-year surgical residency at the Mayo Clinic. Throughout his career, he has received over 40 teaching awards and prizes at the local, state, and national levels, including among the latter the Alpha Omega Alpha Distinguished Professor Award from the Association of American Medical Colleges, and the National Golden Apple from the American Medical Student Association.

In the late 1980s and early 1990s, Dr. Pestana was a member of the Comprehensive Part II Committee of the National Board of Medical Examiners, which designed what is now the clinical component of the Licensure Examination (Step 2 of the USMLE®), and he also served for 8 years as a member-at-large of the National Boards.

For Test Changes or Late-Breaking Developments

KAPTEST.COM/PUBLISHING

The material in this book is up-to-date at the time of publication. However, the Federation of State Medical Boards (FSMB) and the National Board of Medical Examiners (NBME) may have instituted changes in the test after this book was published. Be sure to carefully read the materials you receive when you register for the test. If there are any important late-breaking developments—or any changes or corrections to the Kaplan test preparation materials in this book—we will post that information online at *kaptest.com/publishing*.

For Questions or Feedback About This Book

Contact us at *booksupport@kaplan.com*.

KAPLAN MEDICAL

Preface

The front cover says "Surgery Notes." Your curiosity is aroused: "I always wanted to know how an appendectomy is done. Let me look inside and find out." You will not encounter that information. Surgeons obviously have to know that, but this little book was written for medical students and physicians preparing to take a licensure exam. For those purposes, you have to understand surgical diseases—to know when to operate and which procedure is indicated—but not exactly the technical steps.

Surgeons themselves recognize that the most important thing they do is to choose the *who* and *when* and *what*, rather than the how. Although surgeons take great pride in providing flawless execution, which is of course terribly important, they dismiss it out of hand with the classic joke: "You could teach a monkey how to operate."

But before we leave the operating room, let's look at what goes on in there with a brief historical perspective.

By around 1910, virtually all our surgical armamentarium had been developed, mostly in Western Europe. The last two areas, open-heart surgery and transplantation, were added around the mid-1900s. As they pertained to the two major body cavities, the abdomen and the chest, they were approached via large incisions. That "open" route provided good exposure, allowing the surgeon and assistants to use normal hand motions. Not only could they see what they were doing, but they also could feel the structures being dissected. Stones could be palpated, pulsations detected. When unexpected bleeding arose, direct pressure could instantly stanch it while additional help was summoned. It worked.

But it worked at a price—paid by the patient, as a true story from my days at the Mayo Clinic illustrates. Dr. C. W. Mayo, with his retinue of residents, students, and nurses, was making rounds on a postoperative patient. Pointing to the long, recently sutured abdominal incision, Dr. Mayo praised the virtues of generous access. "Make them big," he said. "They heal from side to side, and not from end to end."

At which point the patient interjected, "Yes, but they hurt from end to end."

Indeed they did. And a laparotomy was not the worst. The traditional approach to the chest, a posterolateral thoracotomy, was the most painful incision that could be inflicted on a human being. Every breath afterward was pure agony.

Unknown to the patients, and mostly ignored by the physicians, was the other cost of those big cuts: They were destructive. The vast majority of metabolic response to trauma often came from the incision itself rather than from what was done inside.

The stage was thus set for the revolution that began in the second half of the 20th century and continues to this day: minimally invasive surgery.

Consider the example of laparoscopic surgery: Carbon dioxide is insufflated into the abdomen to make room to conduct the procedure. A thin tube with a TV camera and a light source—a laparoscope—is introduced through a tiny incision, and the area to be worked on appears on a TV screen. Additional probes are then added through other ports to do the actual operation, with scissors, staplers, cautery tips, and so on, at the working end of those long sticks. Moving these ingenious instruments requires complex, unnatural motions both to position the tip and to activate the various functions—requiring the surgeon and assistants to master new skills of hand-eye coordination.

There is no palpatory input, the image is two-dimensional, and if anything goes wrong the belly has to be opened. In planning for a laparoscopic procedure, it is made clear to the patient that old-fashioned open surgery is the standard. Every effort will be made to complete everything with minimally invasive techniques, but converting to open is not a complication, an error, or an untoward outcome. It is simply the prudent thing to do if needed.

Proprietary developments have improved the basic procedures. More sophisticated setups allow three-dimensional images, with robotic surgery representing the most expensive and elaborate end of the spectrum. In the latter, the surgeon sits at a console wearing gloves that transmit all the hand motions to a tiny robot that has been previously introduced into the patient. In contrast with the forced, awkward motions of laparoscopic surgery, the surgeon uses enhanced natural movements. The robot, for instance, can rotate more than a human hand can. That little device can twist and turn in every desirable way. Like magic.

But even there, surgeon and patient are in the same room. The little robots can do wonders, but human intervention may become necessary if unexpected problems arise.

In the field of vascular surgery, thoracotomies and laparotomies are nowadays often replaced by endovascular procedures, in which a stent is introduced via the femoral artery and then advanced under x-ray guidance and fixed in the location where a major vessel needs to be repaired.

Let's leave the operating room for now, and direct our attention to the contents of these surgery notes. For several decades, I ran a course at the San Antonio medical school that prepared our students to function in the surgical wards and confront their exams. To facilitate those tasks, I wrote a pocket manual for them—a humble, homemade product, distributed at no cost. Somehow, that booklet was posted on the Internet, and to my delighted surprise students all over the nation were downloading and praising it. That was the forerunner of this little book, currently enhanced by the editorial input of Kaplan, and regularly updated.

This is not a substitute for learning "on the job." Your professors, your residents, and your patients will be your best teachers, along with the library, standard textbooks, and your computer. (You just need to remember one word: "Google.") But the clerkship does not expose you to every surgical disease, and there will be times when you need a quick answer. Keep my notes in your white coat, with the lab slips and the granola bars. There is a lot of information in there.

To prove that, let me address an issue that I have never seen covered in any publication or medical school lecture. Surgery is an art, more than a science. There are multiple ways to diagnose and treat patients: regional variations, institutional preferences, evolving criteria. Students are bewildered when they read two different books and are given different advice. They want to know which is the correct answer for the exam.

Let me share a little secret with you. The design features of National Board exams stipulate that any given question can have only one correct answer. The distractors obviously have to be believable, but none of them can be true. Thus, if you read in one book that Disease A should be managed with Therapy X, while another text recommended Therapy Y, you have to remember both therapies. One of them will appear on an item dealing with Disease A—but not both. It's against the rules.

Now let's move to a more sophisticated level of examination, requiring greater discrimination on the exam candidate's part. Here, a prohibition applies to the particular patient described in the stem of the vignette (i.e., it is not a blanket no-no), and the answer options offer both Therapy X and Therapy Y as the right way to take care of "Patient Q." Does this mean that the National

Board of Medical Examiners has made a mistake? No, it does not. Their quality control is awesome. Rather, it signifies that this particular individual has an additional problem precluding the use of one of the proposed answers.

Let's look at an actual example. Go to the back of this book and read question 53. It describes a dissecting aneurysm of the ascending aorta, which can be diagnosed with a sonogram, an MRI, or a CT angiogram. Two of those appear to be correct answers. But the patient in question has a creatinine of 4, indicative of severe kidney disease. Her renal function would be wiped out by the intravenous dye needed to do the CT angio. That would not be good. You have to pick MRI for her.

Which brings us to a little review of those practice questions at the end of the book.

A Note on the Practice Questions

An exam question, from the exam writer's perspective, is designed to conceal the important diagnostic clues among a mass of information that is not particularly relevant to that specific case, thus testing the ability of the well-informed examinee to instantly separate the wheat from the chaff.

The typical exam question always starts with age and gender, followed by present complaint, past history, physical exam, and lab or imaging studies. Each of those "chapters" includes standard data, whether relevant or not. For instance, the vital signs are always given: temperature, pulse rate, blood pressure, height, and weight. In a trauma patient who is in shock, the pulse rate and blood pressure are extremely important. In a woman with a breast mass, they are not. Personal habits are irrelevant in deciding whether somebody has a brain tumor, but would be virtually diagnostic in someone with a neck mass.

By contrast, **the questions in this book are primarily designed for content review,** and are abbreviated versions of the longer, ritualized format of the actual USMLE or shelf exam questions. They are not cluttered with vital signs or other facts that will not help. Rather, **these questions contain only the key combination of facts** that should be immediately recognized by an astute clinician.

A preface typically ends with words of thanks to those who helped with the text. My gratitude extends first of all to my readers, who, by accepting the three previous editions, made this fourth one possible. Then hats off to the faculty at the San Antonio medical school. They helped me teach the surgery course for many years, and they still keep me on my toes. But I mentioned something about regional and institutional preferences, which make this discipline an art rather than a science. So, let me recognize the coast-to-coast contributions of the Kaplan Medical faculty: Dr. Adil Farooqui of Los Angeles; Dr. Mark Nolan Hill of Chicago; and Dr. Ted A. James of Burlington, Vermont.

Carlos Pestana, MD, PhD

San Antonio, Texas

Section I
Surgery Review

Chapter 1

Trauma

Initial Survey (the ABCs)

Airway

An airway is present if the patient is conscious and speaking in a normal tone of voice. The airway will soon be lost if there is an expanding hematoma or emphysema in the neck. An airway should be secured before the situation becomes critical.

An airway is also needed if the patient is unconscious (with a Glasgow Coma Scale of 8 or under) or his breathing is noisy or gurgly, if severe inhalation injury (breathing smoke) has occurred, or if it is necessary to connect the patient to a respirator. If an indication for securing an airway exists in a patient with potential cervical spine injury, the airway has to be secured before dealing with the cervical spine injury.

An airway is most commonly inserted by orotracheal intubation, under direct vision with the use of a laryngoscope, assisted in the awake patient by rapid induction with monitoring of pulse oxymetry, or less commonly with the help of topical anesthesia. In the presence of a cervical spine injury, orotracheal intubation can still be done if the head is secured and not moved. Another option in that setting is nasotracheal intubation over a fiber optic bronchoscope.

The use of a fiberoptic bronchoscope is mandatory when securing an airway if there is subcutaneous emphysema in the neck, which is a sign of major traumatic disruption of the tracheobronchial tree.

If for any reason (laryngospasm, severe maxillofacial injuries, an impacted foreign body that cannot be dislodged, etc.) **intubation cannot be done in the usual manner** and we are running out of time, a cricothyroidotomy may become necessary. It is the quickest and safest way to temporarily gain access before the patient sustains anoxic injury. Because of the potential need for future laryngeal reconstruction, however, we are reluctant to do it before the age of 12.

Breathing

Hearing breath sounds on both sides of the chest and having satisfactory pulse oximetry establishes that breathing is okay.

Shock

Clinical signs of shock include low blood pressure (BP) (under 90 mm Hg systolic), fast feeble pulse, and low urinary output (under 0.5 mL/kg/h) in a patient who is pale, cold, shivering, sweating, thirsty, and apprehensive.

In the trauma setting, shock is caused by either bleeding (hypovolemic-hemorrhagic, by far the most common cause), pericardial tamponade, or tension pneumothorax. For either of the last two to occur, there must be trauma to the chest (blunt or penetrating). In shock caused by bleeding, the central venous pressure (CVP) is low (empty veins clinically). In both pericardial tamponade and tension pneumothorax, CVP is high (big distended head and neck veins clinically). In pericardial tamponade there is no respiratory distress. In tension pneumothorax there is severe respiratory distress, one side of the chest has no breath sounds and is hyperresonant to percussion, and the mediastinum is displaced to the opposite side (tracheal deviation).

The treatment of hemorrhagic shock in the urban setting (big trauma center nearby), with penetrating injuries that will require surgery anyway, starts with the surgical intervention to stop the bleeding, and volume replacement takes place afterward. In all other settings, volume replacement is the first step, starting with about 2 L of Ringer lactate (without sugar), followed by packed red cells, fresh frozen plasma, and platelet packs, in a 1-1-1 ratio until urinary output reaches 0.5 to 2 mL/kg/h, while not exceeding CVP of 15 mm Hg.

Massive Bleeding

Uncontrolled massive bleeding is lethal, and so is untreated hemorrhagic shock.

In the usual civilian setting, where one single patient arrives with a visible source of bleeding to an ER staffed by tons of people, that bleeding is best controlled with local pressure. A gloved finger pushes and occludes the lacerated vessel until it can be repaired.

In the military setting, where 10 soldiers may be blown up by a roadside bomb and there is only one medic to look after them, the obvious life-savers are tourniquets. The same is true in massive civilian casualties. When terrorists deploy explosives that maim dozens of people lined up watching a parade, the first responders also have to resort to tourniquets as they sort out and transport the victims.

Once bleeding is controlled, hemorrhagic shock, if present, has to be dealt with. The obvious final therapy for lost whole blood, is whole blood. The military often can do that. All soldiers have been typed, are certified not to have blood-borne diseases, and are typically willing to donate blood to their injured comrades. But in the civilian world we can't ask for whole blood. Blood is a scarce resource, and blood banks break it down into components to make more efficient use of it. If we want whole blood, we have to reconstitute it by the 1-1-1 expedient already mentioned.

Preferred route of fluid resuscitation in the trauma setting is 2 peripheral IV lines, 16-gauge. If they cannot be inserted, percutaneous femoral vein catheter or saphenous vein cut-downs are alternatives. In children under 6 years of age, intraosseus cannulation of the proximal tibia is the alternate route.

Management of pericardial tamponade is based on clinical diagnosis (do not order x-rays—if diagnosis is unclear choose sonogram), and centered on prompt evacuation of the pericardial sac (by pericardiocentesis, tube, pericardial window, or open thoracotomy). Fluid and blood administration while evacuation is being set up is helpful.

Management of tension pneumothorax is also based on clinical diagnosis (do not order x-rays or wait for blood gases). Start with big needle or big IV catheter into the affected pleural space. Follow with chest tube connected to underwater seal (both inserted high in the anterior chest wall).

Brief detour: Shock in the nontrauma setting

Shock can be hypovolemic, from bleeding or other massive fluid loss (burns, pancreatitis, severe diarrhea). The classical clinical signs of shock will include a low CVP. Treat the cause, and replace the volume.

Intrinsic cardiogenic shock can happen with massive infarction or fulminating myocarditis. In this case the clinical signs will come with a high CVP, a key identifying feature. Treat with circulatory support.

Vasomotor shock is seen in anaphylactic reactions and high spinal cord transection or high spinal anesthetic. Circulatory collapse occurs in flushed, "pink and warm" patient. CVP is low. Pharmacologic treatment to restore peripheral resistance is the main therapy (vasopressors). Additional fluids will help.

Septic shock includes all three components. Early on, low peripheral resistance and high cardiac output predominate. Later, cardiogenic and hypovolemic features are seen. In addition to antibiotics, the initial treatment often includes a steroid bolus. Patients who respond beautifully at first but then suffer a relapse might not have septic shock at all, but rather **adrenal insufficiency**. It is not common, but you will look very smart if you make that diagnosis.

A Review from Head to Toe

Head Trauma

Penetrating head trauma as a rule requires surgical intervention and repair of the damage.

Linear skull fractures are left alone if they are closed (no overlying wound). Open fractures require wound closure. If comminuted or depressed, they have to be treated in the operating room (OR).

Anyone with head trauma who has become unconscious gets a computed tomography (CT) scan to look for intracranial hematomas. If negative and neurologically intact, they can go home if the family will wake them up frequently during the next 24 hours to make sure they are not going into coma.

Signs of a fracture affecting the base of the skull include raccoon eyes, rhinorrhea, and otorrhea or ecchymosis behind the ear. Expectant management is the rule. From our perspective, the significance of a base of the skull fracture is that it indicates that the patient sustained very severe head trauma, and thus it requires that we assess the integrity of the cervical spine. This is best done with CT scan, usually as an extension of the scan that is done for the head. Remember also that nasal endotracheal intubation should be avoided in these patients.

Neurologic damage from trauma can be caused by 3 components: the initial blow, the subsequent development of a hematoma that displaces the midline structures, and the later development of increased intracranial pressure (ICP). There is no treatment for the first, surgery can relieve the second, and medical measures can prevent or minimize the third.

Acute epidural hematoma occurs with modest trauma to the side of the head and has classic sequence of trauma, unconsciousness, lucid interval (with completely asymptomatic patient who returns to his previous activity), gradual lapsing into coma again, fixed dilated pupil (90% of the time on the side of the hematoma), and contralateral hemiparesis with decerebrate posture. CT scan shows biconvex, lens-shaped hematoma. Emergency craniotomy produces dramatic cure. Because every patient who has been unconscious gets CT scan, the full-blown picture with the fixed pupil and the contralateral hemiparesis is seldom seen.

Acute subdural hematoma has the same sequence, but the trauma is much bigger, the patient is usually much sicker (not fully awake and asymptomatic at any point), and the neurologic damage is severe (because of the initial blow). CT scan will show semilunar, crescent-shaped hematoma. If midline structures are deviated, craniotomy will help, but prognosis is bad. If there is no deviation, therapy is centered on preventing further damage from subsequent increased ICP. Do ICP monitoring, elevate head, hyperventilate, avoid fluid overload, and give mannitol or furosemide. Do not diurese to the point of lowering systemic arterial pressure. (Brain perfusion = arterial pressure – intracranial pressure.) Hyperventilation is recommended when there are signs of herniation, and the goal is a PCO_2 of 35. Sedation and hypothermia have been used to decrease brain activity and oxygen demand. Hypothermia is currently suggested as a better option to reduce oxygen demand. As an interesting aside, we will encounter the topic of increased intracranial pressure again when we review brain tumors. We treat that problem with high-dose steroids, rather than in the way we have just detailed in cases of trauma.

Diffuse axonal injury occurs in more severe trauma. CT scan shows diffuse blurring of the gray-white matter interface and multiple small punctate hemorrhages. Without hematoma there is no role for surgery. Therapy is directed at preventing further damage from increased ICP.

Chronic subdural hematoma occurs in the very old or in severe alcoholics. A shrunken brain is rattled around the head by minor trauma, tearing venous sinuses. Over several days or weeks, mental function deteriorates as hematoma forms. CT scan is diagnostic, and surgical evacuation provides dramatic cure.

Hypovolemic shock cannot happen from intracranial bleeding. There isn't enough space inside the head for the amount of blood loss needed to produce shock. Look for another source.

Neck Trauma

Penetrating trauma to the neck leads to surgical exploration in all cases where there is an expanding hematoma, deteriorating vital signs, or clear signs of esophageal or tracheal injury (coughing or spitting up blood). A strong tradition of surgical exploration for all gunshot wounds of the middle zone of the neck (regardless of symptoms) is giving way to a more selective approach.

More selective approaches in other settings include the following: for gunshot wounds to the **upper zone,** arteriographic diagnosis and management is preferred; for gunshot wounds to the **base of the neck,** arteriography, esophagogram (water-soluble, followed by barium if negative), esophagoscopy, and bronchoscopy before surgery help decide the specific surgical approach.

Stab wounds to the upper and middle zones in asymptomatic patients can be safely observed.

In all patients with severe blunt trauma to the neck, the integrity of the cervical spine has to be ascertained. If there are neurologic deficits, the need to radiologically exam the neck with a CT scan of the cervical spine is obvious, but it also has to be done in neurologically intact patients who have pain to local palpation over the cervical spine. In the emergency department setting, CT scan is the best way to assess the status of the cervical spine. If a CT of the head is ordered secondary to head trauma, this scan can be extended to include the neck.

Spinal Cord Injuries

Complete transection is unlikely to be on the exam because it is too easy: Nothing works (sensory or motor) below the lesion.

Hemisection (Brown-Séquard) is typically from clean-cut injury (knife blade) and has paralysis and loss of proprioception distal to the injury on the injury side and loss of pain perception distal to the injury on the other side.

Anterior cord syndrome is typically seen in burst fractures of the vertebral bodies. There is loss of motor function and loss of pain and temperature sensation on both sides distal to the injury, with preservation of vibratory and positional sense.

Central cord syndrome occurs in the elderly with forced hyperextension of the neck (rear-end collision). There is paralysis and burning pain in the upper extremities, with preservation of most functions in the lower extremities.

Management: Precise diagnosis of cord injury is best done with magnetic resonance imaging (MRI; CT is easier to do if we only have to look at the bone). The use of corticosteroids immediately after the injury is no longer recommended. Further surgical management is too specialized for our level of review.

Chest Trauma

Rib fracture can be deadly in the elderly, because of progression of pain → hypoventilation → atelectasis → pneumonia. Treat with local nerve block and epidural catheter.

Plain pneumothorax results from penetrating trauma (which could be the jagged edge of a broken rib or any of the more common penetrating weapons). There is moderate shortness of breath, and one side of the thorax has no breath sounds and is hyperresonant to percussion. Get chest x-ray, place chest tube (upper, anterior), and connect to underwater seal.

Hemothorax happens the same way, but affected side will be dull to percussion. It is diagnosed by chest x-ray. Blood needs to be evacuated to prevent development of empyema, thus chest tube (placed low) is needed, but surgery to stop the bleeding is seldom required. The lung is the usual bleeding source, and it will stop by itself (low pressure system). If we get 1,500 mL or more of blood when the chest tube is inserted (or more than 600 mL is collected in the ensuing 6 hours), we realize that a systemic vessel is lacerated. This is typically an intercostal artery, and video-assisted thoracotomy will be needed to control the bleeding.

In severe blunt trauma to the chest there may be obvious injuries, plus hidden injuries. The latter have to be monitored for (blood gases and chest x-ray to detect developing pulmonary contusion; cardiac enzymes [troponins] and electrocardiogram [EKG] to detect myocardial contusion) or actively sought at the outset (traumatic transection of the aorta).

Sucking chest wounds are obvious from physical exam, as there is a flap that sucks air with inspiration and closes during expiration. Untreated, it will lead to deadly tension pneumothorax. First aid is with occlusive dressing that allows air out (taped on 3 sides) but not in.

Flail chest occurs with multiple rib fractures that allow a segment of the chest wall to cave in during inspiration and bulge out during expiration (paradoxic breathing). The real problem is the underlying pulmonary contusion. Contused lung is very sensitive to fluid overload, thus treatment includes fluid restriction and use of diuretics. Pulmonary dysfunction may develop, thus blood gases have to be monitored. If a respirator is needed, bilateral chest tubes are advisable to prevent tension pneumothorax from developing (the multiple broken ribs may have punctured the lung). To get a flail chest big trauma is required, thus traumatic transection of the aorta must be actively sought.

Pulmonary contusion can show up right away after chest trauma, with deteriorating blood gases and "white out" of the lungs on chest x-ray, or it can appear up to 48 hours later (thus it is one of those hidden injuries that has to be monitored for). Treatment as detailed above for flail chest.

Myocardial contusion should be suspected in sternal fractures. EKG monitoring will detect it. Troponins are quite specific. Treatment is focused on the complications, such as arrhythmias.

Traumatic rupture of the diaphragm shows up with bowel in the chest (by physical exam and x-rays), always on the left side. All suspicious cases should be evaluated with laparoscopy. Surgical repair is typically done from the abdomen.

Traumatic rupture of the aorta is the ultimate "hidden injury." It happens at the junction of the arch and the descending aorta, requires big deceleration injury, and is totally asymptomatic until the hematoma contained by the adventitia blows up and kills the patient. Suspicion should be triggered by the mechanism of injury (knowing that the patient suffered severe deceleration injury) or by the presence of fractures in chest bones that are "very hard to break": first rib, scapula, or sternum, or by the presence of wide mediastinum. Noninvasive diagnostic tests include: transesophageal echocardiography, spiral CT scan, or MRI angiography. In the trauma setting, the most practical of these is the spiral CT scan, which is enhanced by intravenous dye, and thus is also known as CT angio. As in other areas of vascular surgery, repair of these is now done, whenever possible, with endovascular prosthesis rather than open thoracotomy.

Traumatic rupture of the trachea or major bronchus is suggested by developing subcutaneous emphysema in the upper chest and lower neck, or by a large "air leak" from a chest tube. Chest x-ray confirms the presence of air in the tissues, and fiberoptic bronchoscopy identifies the lesion and allows intubation to secure an airway beyond the lesion. Surgical repair follows.

Differential diagnosis of subcutaneous emphysema also includes rupture of the esophagus (but the usual setting is after endoscopy) and tension pneumothorax (but in the latter the other findings— shock and respiratory distress—are far more alarming and deadly).

Air embolism should be suspected when sudden death occurs in a chest trauma patient who is intubated and on a respirator. It also happens when the subclavian vein is opened to the air (supraclavicular node biopsies, central venous line placement, CVP lines that become disconnected), also leading to sudden collapse and cardiac arrest. Immediate management includes cardiac massage, with the patient positioned with the left side down. Prevention includes the Trendelenburg position when the great veins at the base of the neck are to be entered.

Fat embolism may be seen in multiple trauma patients with several long bone fractures. They develop petechial rashes in the axillae and neck; present with fever, tachycardia, and low platelet count; and eventually become a full-blown picture of respiratory distress with hypoxemia and bilateral patchy infiltrates on chest x-ray. Treatment is respiratory support using a respirator. Rarely, fat droplets may reach the brain, producing unexpected coma. A "star-field pattern" on MRI is diagnostic. Spontaneous resolution is possible, and thus one should not rush to declare irreversible damage and withdraw further care.

Abdominal Trauma

Gunshot wounds to the abdomen require exploratory laparotomy for repair of intraabdominal injuries (not necessarily to "remove the bullet"). Any entrance or exit wound below the level of the nipple line is considered to involve the abdomen. In very select cases of abdominal trauma due to low caliber gunshot wounds involving the right upper quadrant, conservative therapy may be used if the patient is properly monitored with close follow-up of clinical signs and serial abdominal CT scans.

Stab wounds allow a more individualized approach. If it is clear that penetration has occurred (protruding viscera), exploratory laparotomy is mandatory. The same is true if hemodynamic instability or signs of peritoneal irritation develop. In the absence of the above, digital exploration of the wound in the ER (gentle insertion of gloved finger) and observation may be sufficient. If digital exploration is equivocal, a CT scan is diagnostic.

Blunt trauma to the abdomen requires exploratory laparotomy if signs of peritoneal irritation (an acute abdomen) develop. Otherwise, in blunt trauma one must determine whether there are internal injuries, whether there is bleeding into the peritoneal cavity, and whether the bleeding is likely to stop by itself or will require surgical intervention. The finding that triggers such investigation is the presence of signs of internal bleeding (patient going into shock, with low CVP, with no obvious external source of blood loss).

Signs of internal bleeding in a patient with blunt trauma include a drop in blood pressure, with fast thready pulse, low CVP, and low urinary output, in a cold, pale, anxious patient who is shivering, thirsty, and perspiring profusely. Those signs of shock occur when 25–30% of blood volume is acutely lost (about 1,500 mL in the average size adult), and thus there are few places within the body where such large amounts of blood could hide. It cannot do it in the head (a much smaller amount would produce lethal neurologic damage by compression and displacement of the brain). The neck could accommodate a large hematoma, but gross deformity would be obvious on physical exam. Blood in the pericardial sac would lead to pericardial tamponade. The pleural cavities could easily accommodate several liters of blood, with relatively few local symptoms, but that blood could not hide from an x-ray machine (a few hundred milliliters show up on chest x-ray). By virtue of their size, the arms and lower legs would also show gross deformity if they were the site of a 1,500-mL hematoma. That leaves the abdomen, thighs (secondary to femur fractures), and pelvis (in pelvic fractures) as the only 3 places where 1,500 mL of blood could "hide" in a blunt trauma patient who has developed shock. The femurs and pelvis are always checked for fractures in the initial survey of the trauma patient (by physical exam, with x-rays if needed). So, the multiple trauma patient who has a normal chest x-ray and no evidence of pelvic or femur fracture has to be suspected of intraabdominal bleeding when he or she goes into hypovolemic shock for no obvious reason. This has to be proven, because the blood loss might have been to the outside, rather than internal.

The diagnosis of intraabdominal bleeding can be made most accurately with CT scan. CT will show the presence of blood, will show the injury from where the blood is coming (most frequently liver or spleen), and will even give an idea of how bad that injury is. In conjunction with the patient's response to fluid administration, it allows a decision to be made for surgery or expectant therapy. The patient with minor internal injuries who responds promptly to fluid resuscitation does not need surgery. The patient with major injuries and vital signs that do not improve with fluid resuscitation will require surgery. Even though fast CT scanners are available in Level I trauma centers, it is imperative that the patient be hemodynamically stable so that pictures can be taken without all the commotion of continuing resuscitation efforts.

The diagnosis of intraabdominal bleeding in the patient who is hemodynamically unstable has to be made quickly in the ER or OR, at the same time that resuscitation efforts are under way. This is best done with a limited sonogram, known by the acronym FAST (Focused Abdominal Sonogram for Trauma). The test simply confirms that the belly is full of blood, and prompt laparotomy will ensue. (FAST has already displaced the older, invasive, diagnostic peritoneal lavage.)

A ruptured spleen is the most common source of significant intraabdominal bleeding in blunt abdominal trauma. (If all patients are counted—significant and insignificant—the liver is a more common source.) Often there are additional diagnostic hints, such as fractures of lower ribs on the left side. Given the immunologic function of the spleen, every effort will be made to repair it rather than remove it—particularly in children. If removal is unavoidable (truly smashed to pieces, or there are many other life-threatening injuries that preclude the use of operative time for repair), postoperative immunization against encapsulated bacteria is mandatory (Pneumococcus, *Haemophilus influenza* B, and meningococcus).

Intraoperative development of coagulopathy during prolonged abdominal surgery for multiple trauma with multiple transfusions is treated empirically with platelet packs and fresh-frozen plasma, approximately 10 units of each. If in addition to coagulopathy there is hypothermia and acidosis, the laparotomy has to be promptly terminated, with packing of bleeding surfaces and temporary closure. The operation can be resumed later when the patient has been warmed and the coagulopathy treated.

The abdominal compartment syndrome occurs when lots of fluids and blood have been given during the course of prolonged laparotomies, so that by the time of closure all the tissues are swollen and the abdominal wound cannot be closed without undue tension. In those cases, a temporary cover is placed over the abdominal contents, either an absorbable mesh (that can later be grafted over) or nonabsorbable plastic to be removed at a later date when closure might be possible. This syndrome may not be evident until the second postoperative day in a patient on whom closure was done; who subsequently goes on to develop distention, with the sutures cutting through the tissues, hypoxia secondary to inability to breathe, and renal failure from the pressure on the vena cava. In that setting, the abdomen must be opened and a temporary cover provided.

Damage control laparotomy has become the standard concept that now guides management of the severely traumatized patient, who is subject to consumption coagulopathy, hypothermia, and the abdominal compartment syndrome. These patients can now be identified ahead of time, as surgeons have gained experience with their management. The operation is designed, up front, to be brief. Clamp all the bleeders, temporarily occlude damaged viscera, clean up all the contamination, and get out of there. Then do the rest of the resuscitation, and at a later date go back in and finish the job.

Pelvic Fractures

Pelvic hematomas are typically left alone if they are not expanding.

In any pelvic fracture, associated injuries have to be ruled out. These include rectum (do rectal exam and proctoscopy) and bladder (more about that later) in both sexes; and vagina in women (do pelvic exam); or urethra in men (do retrograde urethrogram).

Pelvic fractures can be the site of significant, potentially deadly hemorrhage. We realize that is happening when we see signs of hypovolemic shock in a trauma patient who has a pelvic fracture with a big hematoma, and no evidence of bleeding anywhere else. This problem does not have a surgical solution. The site of blood loss is often inaccessible and not amenable to clamping or electrocoagulation. We rely instead on two things: immobilizing the pelvis as best we can, and angiographic management. We do the first with binding or external fixation and the second with embolization of either specific bleeding arteries or of internal iliacs to minimize venous bleeding.

Urologic Injuries

The hallmark of urologic injuries is blood in the urine in someone who has sustained penetrating or blunt abdominal trauma. Gross hematuria in that setting must be investigated with appropriate studies.

Penetrating urologic injuries are as a rule surgically explored and repaired.

Blunt urologic injuries may affect the kidney, in which case the associated injuries tend to be lower rib fractures. If they affect the bladder or urethra, the usual associated injury is pelvic fracture.

Urethral injury occurs almost exclusively in men, is typically associated with a pelvic fracture, and may present with blood at the meatus.

More complete clinical picture might include a scrotal hematoma, for posterior injuries the sensation of wanting to void but not being able to do it, and a "high-riding" prostate on rectal exam. The key issue in any of those is that a Foley catheter should not be inserted (it might compound an existing injury), but a retrograde urethrogram should be done instead. If by chance someone had attempted to pass a Foley catheter and met resistance, that would be another diagnostic clue suggesting urethral injury.

Bladder injuries can occur in either sex, are usually associated with pelvic fracture, and are diagnosed by retrograde cystogram. The x-ray study must include postvoid films, to see extraperitoneal leaks at the base of the bladder that might be obscured by the bladder full of dye. If the latter are found, they can be treated simply by placing a Foley catheter. For intraperitoneal leaks, surgical repair is done and protected with a suprapubic cystostomy.

Renal injuries secondary to blunt trauma are usually associated with lower rib fractures. They are assessed by CT scan, and most of the time can be managed without surgical intervention. A rare but fascinating potential sequela of injuries affecting the renal pedicle is the development of an arteriovenous fistula leading to congestive heart failure. Should renal artery stenosis develop after trauma, renovascular hypertension is another potential sequela.

Scrotal hematomas can attain alarming size but typically do not need specific intervention unless the testicle is ruptured. The latter can be assessed with sonogram.

Fracture of the penis (fracture of the corpora cavernosa, fracture of the tunica albuginea) occurs to an erect penis, typically as an accident during vigorous intercourse (with woman on top). There is sudden pain and development of a large penile shaft hematoma, with a normal-appearing glans. Frequently, the true history will be concealed by an embarrassed patient who concocts a cover story (the toilet seat lid fell on him, or some such thing). Emergency surgical repair is required. If not done, impotence will ensue as arteriovenous shunts will develop.

The Extremities

In penetrating injuries of the extremities, the main issue is whether a vascular injury has occurred or not. Anatomic location provides the first clue. When there are no major vessels in the vicinity of the injury tract, only tetanus prophylaxis and cleaning of the wound is required. If the penetration is near major vessels and the patient is asymptomatic, Doppler studies or CT angio are done. If there is an obvious vascular injury (absent distal pulses, expanding hematoma), surgical exploration and repair are required.

Combined injuries of arteries, nerves, and bone obviously need repair, but they pose the challenge of which one to do first. The usual sequence is to stabilize the bone first, then do the delicate vascular repair (which would be otherwise disrupted by the rough handling needed to put together a bone), and leave the nerve for last. A fasciotomy should be added because the prolonged ischemia could lead to a compartment syndrome.

High-velocity gunshot wounds (military or big-game hunting rifles) produce a large cone of tissue destruction that requires extensive debridements and potential amputations.

Crushing injuries of the extremities pose the hazard of hyperkalemia, myoglobinemia, myoglobinuria, and renal failure, as well as potential development of compartment syndrome. For the first, vigorous fluid administration, osmotic diuretics, and alkalinization of the urine are good preventive measures. For the latter, a fasciotomy may be required.

Burns

Chemical burns require massive irrigation to remove the offending agent. Alkaline burns (Liquid Plumr, Drano) are worse than acid burns (battery acid). Irrigation must begin as soon as possible at the site where the injury occurred (tap water, shower). Do not "play chemist" and attempt to neutralize the agent.

High-voltage electrical burns are always deeper and worse than they appear to be. Massive debridements or amputations may be required. Additional concerns include myoglobinemia-myoglobinuria-renal failure (give plenty of fluids and osmotic diuretics like mannitol, and alkalinize the urine), orthopedic injuries secondary to massive muscle contractions (posterior dislocation of the shoulder, compression fractures of vertebral bodies), and late development of cataracts and demyelinization syndromes.

Respiratory burns (inhalation injuries) occur with flame burns in an enclosed space (a burning building, car, plane) and are chemical injuries caused by smoke inhalation. Burns around the mouth or soot inside the throat are suggestive clues. Diagnosis is confirmed with fiberoptic bronchoscopy, but the key issue is whether respiratory support (a respirator) is needed or not, and blood gases are best to make that determination. Intubation should be done if there is any concern about adequacy of the airway. The level of carboxyhemoglobin must be monitored. If elevated, 100% oxygen will shorten its half-life.

Circumferential burns of the extremities can lead to cutoff of the blood supply as edema accumulates underneath the unyielding eschar. In circumferential burns of the chest, a similar mechanical problem may interfere with breathing. Escharotomies (done at the bedside, with no need for anesthesia) will provide immediate relief.

Scalding burns in children should always raise the suspicion of child abuse, particularly if the pattern of the burn does not fit the description of the event given by the parents. A classic example is burns of both buttocks, which are typically produced by holding a small child by arms and legs, and dunking him into boiling water.

Fluid replacement in the severely burned patient is the most critical, life-saving component of the management of extensive thermal burns. Underneath a deep burn, a lot of fluid accumulates. This is essentially plasma that has been temporarily lost from the circulating space and trapped at the burn site. In extensive burns, this internal shift of fluids is enormous and, if untreated, leads to hypovolemic shock and death. Thus, large infusions of intravenous fluids are required.

Complicated formulas were devised to estimate how much fluid would be needed. They multiplied the weight of the patient in kilograms by the extent of the burn as a percentage of body surface (capped at 50%; beyond that there is no further fluid loss). The involved body surface was calculated by the "rule of 9s," assigning 9% of body surface to the head and to each upper extremity, double that to each lower extremity, and 4 times that much to the trunk. The product was then multiplied by another number, empirically arrived at, ranging between 4 and 6, depending on the specific formula. That final calculation gave us milliliters of Ringer lactate that were meant to be infused most rapidly in the first 8 hours, tapering afterwards, and supplemented by a couple of liters of D5W every day and, if desired, by colloids on the second day. The expectation was that no fluids would be needed by the third day, when the plasma trapped in the burn edema would be reabsorbed and a large diuresis would ensue.

In reality, most of these complicated calculations and instructions were never carried out: As soon as hourly urinary output was available, the therapy was fine-tuned based on the patient's response, aiming for an hourly urinary output of 1 or 2 mL/kg/h, while avoiding CVP over 15 mm Hg. Furthermore, those detailed formulas too often failed to provide accurate numbers. As a result, they have been mostly abandoned in favor of a simpler approach in which fluid infusion is begun at an arbitrary, predetermined rate and then adjusted as needed.

An appropriate predetermined rate of fluid infusion in the adult is to start at 1,000 mL/h of Ringer lactate (without sugar) on anyone whose burns exceed 20% of body surface, and then adjust as needed to produce the desired urinary output. (Sugar is avoided in the Ringer lactate so as not to induce an osmotic diuresis from glycosuria, which would invalidate the meaning of the hourly urinary output.)

Estimation of fluid needs in burned babies differs from the adult in several measures. Babies have bigger heads and smaller legs; thus the "rule of 9s" for them assigns two 9s to the head, and both legs share a total of three 9s instead of four. In determining what is third-degree, we should remember that in babies those areas look deep bright red (rather than the leathery, dry, gray appearance in the adult). Babies need proportionally more fluid than the adult. An appropriate rate of initial fluid administration is 20 mL/kg/h if the burn exceeds 20% of body surface, to be subsequently fine-tuned in response to urinary output.

Other aspects of burn care include tetanus prophylaxis, cleaning of the burn areas, and use of topical agents. The standard topical agent is silver sulfadiazine. If deep penetration is desired (thick eschar, cartilage), mafenide acetate is the choice (do not use it everywhere else; it hurts and it can produce acidosis). Burns near the eyes are covered with triple antibiotic ointment (silver sulfadiazine is irritating to the eyes). In the early period, all pain medication is given intravenously. After an initial day or two of NG suction, intensive nutritional support is provided, preferably via the gut, with high-calorie/high-nitrogen diets. After 2 or 3 weeks of wound care and general support, the burned areas that have not regenerated are grafted. Rehabilitation starts on day one.

The concept of early excision and grafting is used whenever possible to save costs and minimize pain, suffering, and complications. It implies removal in the OR (on day one) of the burned areas, with immediate skin grafting. This can be done only for fairly limited burns (under 20%) that are obviously third-degree, but the experts are extending the concept to highly selected patients with more extensive burns. On an exam question, you can expect the candidate for early excision and grafting to have a very limited burn.

Bites and Stings

Tetanus prophylaxis and wound care are required for all bites.

Dog bites are considered provoked if the dog was petted while eating or otherwise teased. No rabies prophylaxis is required, other than observation of the dog for developing signs of rabies. Because bites to the face are very close to the brain, it might be prudent to start immunization and then discontinue it if observation of the dog is reassuring.

Unprovoked dog bites or bites from wild animals raise the issue of potential rabies. If the animal is available, it can be killed and the brain examined for signs of rabies. Otherwise, rabies prophylaxis is mandatory (immunoglobulin plus vaccine).

Snakebites by crotalids (rattlesnakes) do not necessarily result in envenomation, even if the snake is poisonous (up to 30% of bitten patients are not envenomated). The most reliable signs of envenomation are severe local pain, swelling, and discoloration developing within 30 minutes of the bite. If present, draw blood for typing and crossmatch (they cannot be done later if needed), coagulation studies, and liver and renal function. Treatment is based on antivenin. The currently preferred agent for crotalids is CROFAB, of which several vials are usually needed.

Antivenin dosage relates to size of the envenomation, not size of the patient (children get the same dosages as adults). Surgical excision of the bite site or fasciotomy are very rarely needed. The only valid first aid is to splint the extremity during transportation. All the first aid measures that you learned at boy scouts are wrong. Do not make cruciate cuts, suck out venom, wrap with ice, or apply a tourniquet.

Brightly colored **coral snakes** have a neurotoxin that needs to be promptly neutralized with specific antivenin. Don't wait for signs of envenomation. True coral snakes are identified by the mnemonic

"Red on yellow, kill a fellow," meaning that red rings and yellow rings touch each other. Harmless brightly colored imitators have black rings separating yellow and red.

Bee stings kill many more people in the United States than snakebites because of an anaphylactic reaction. Wheezing and rash may occur, and hypotension when present is caused by vasomotor shock ("pink and warm" shock). Epinephrine is the drug of choice (0.3 to 0.5 mL of 1:1,000 solution). The stingers should be removed without squeezing them.

Black widow spiders are black, with a red hourglass on their belly. Bitten patients get nausea, vomiting, and severe generalized muscle cramps. The antidote is IV calcium gluconate. Muscle relaxants also help.

Brown recluse spider bites are often not recognized at the time. By the next day a skin ulcer develops, with necrotic center and a surrounding halo of erythema. Dapsone is helpful. Surgical excision may be needed but should be delayed until the full extent of the damage is evident (as much as one week). Skin grafting may be needed.

Human bites are bacteriologically the dirtiest bite one can get. They require extensive irrigation and debridement (in the OR). A classic human bite is the sharp cut over the knuckles on someone who punched someone else in the mouth and was cut by the teeth of the victim. They often show up in the ER with a cover story but should be recognized because they need specialized orthopedic care.

Surgical Infections

Infections often occur as an aftermath of the violation of the integrity of the human body, such as trauma. They obviously can also occur as a consequence of disease—for instance, perforation of the colon with subsequent spillage of bacteria into the peritoneal cavity. Many general principles apply to both situations. Let us review them.

When harmful organisms invade our tissues, the ultimate outcome depends on the balance between the virulence of the bugs and the robustness of the body's natural defenses. The principal factor on the side of the invaders is their number; a wound sustained on a battlefield, for instance, starts with a huge inoculum. The second factor in microbes' favor is time. Bacteria in an environment with ideal nutrients, humidity, and temperature multiply at an astonishing speed. Thus, what might begin as a minor contamination—such as a stab wound in a clean setting—will eventually become a real problem if not promptly treated. The "magic" time for that undesirable development is around 6 hours.

On the side of patient, the main defense is the richness of the blood supply at the site of the battle. Well-supplied sites like the face and the soft tissues of the oral cavity get infected very rarely. At the other end of the spectrum are bones, cartilage, and previously irradiated tissues. The bugs typically win there, sometimes helped by systemic conditions like an immunosuppressed state or diabetes.

So, what can we do to help the patient? Bearing in mind what we have reviewed so far, several strategies should be obvious.

Let's start with time: Don't allow those evil bugs to multiply inside the human victim. An individual with a perforated colon or a broken femur sticking out of a dirty wound deserves priority in the scheduling of available operating rooms. Simple mechanical cleansing in the OR will diminish the number of invaders. The

(continued)

Surgical Infections (*Cont'd*)

first order of business is elimination of foreign material and dead tissue, along with massive irrigation: Dilution is the solution to the problem of pollution.

Next, let's look at blood supply: Given its importance, wouldn't it be nice to increase it to tilt the balance in favor of the patient? We can do it with an old trick that is cheap and easy to apply. Consider subcutaneous tissue, another poorly irrigated area of the body.

If we close a heavily contaminated wound, that fatty layer will predictably become an abscess. But if we leave it open, the healing process covers that exposed fat with granulation tissue, which is made up of vascular buds.

Medical students are often bewildered at the end of an operation for a perforated colon when the surgeon tells the chief resident, "Leave the wound open." They have visions of bowel spilling out and flies landing for a drink of blood. What the chief is actually communicating is "Close everything up to and including the fascia, but leave the subcutaneous tissue and skin open." Several days later, when granulation tissue is well established, we can close that wound with impunity.

More recently, we have discovered another way to keep wounds clean: suction. Constant, gentle suction applied by patented mechanical devices has become a common adjuvant in the management of these patients.

What about antibiotics? Aren't they our most potent weapons to kill bacteria?

Yes, antibiotics have a role, but they are not a substitute for the universally applicable measures already discussed. There is no "universal" antibiotic—no single drug or drug combination that can wipe out all harmful bugs. It is beyond the scope of this little book to engage in a detailed discussion of antibiotic choices: More than 150 options are available, and mastery of that topic requires

(continued)

Surgical Infections (*Cont'd*)

a 2-year fellowship beyond basic residency training. We will just mention a couple of examples.

Colonic contents represent one end the spectrum, requiring a combination of agents to cover gram-positive, gram-negative, and anaerobic organisms. Some practitioners use ciprofloxacin and metronidazole in the management of lower GI injury or disease, while some prefer piperacillin and tazobactam and others include imipenem. Skin flora, on the other hand, is typically handled with a single drug. When you first venture into the operating room for a clean, elective case, you will find that surgeons want the patient to have good blood levels of cefazolin during the operation. To ensure this, they administer it 2 hours prior to making the incision.

Many of the rituals of surgery are, in fact, based on the principles that we have just discussed. Because morning hours are very busy in the surgical suite, we used to shave the operating area the night before. No longer. Razor blades can nick the skin and allow bacteria in. Given 12 hours in a warm, moist, nutrient-rich environment, what do those little creatures do? You know: They multiply like crazy. So, now we get rid of the hair just before we prep the area—and we do it with clippers.

Chapter 2
Orthopedics

Disorders in Children

Disorders of the Hip

Developmental dysplasia of the hip runs in families and ideally should be diagnosed right after birth. Children have uneven gluteal folds, and physical examination of the hips shows that they can be easily dislocated posteriorly with a jerk and a "click," and returned to normal with a "snapping." If signs are equivocal, sonogram is diagnostic (do not order x-rays; the hip is not calcified in the newborn). Treatment is abduction splinting with Pavlik harness for about 6 months.

Hip pathology in children may show up with hip pain, or it may show up with knee pain.

Legg-Calvé-Perthes disease (avascular necrosis of the capital femoral epiphysis) occurs around age 6, with insidious development of limping, decreased hip motion, and hip (or knee) pain. Kids walk with an antalgic gait, and passive motion of the hip is guarded. Diagnosis is provided by AP and lateral hip x-rays. Treatment is controversial, usually containing the femoral head within the acetabulum by casting and crutches.

Slipped capital femoral epiphysis is an orthopedic emergency. The typical patient is a chubby (or lanky) boy, around age 13. They complain of groin (or knee) pain and are noted to be limping. When they sit with the legs dangling, the sole of the foot on the affected side points toward the other foot. On physical exam there is limited hip motion, and as the hip is flexed the thigh goes into external rotation and cannot be rotated internally. X-rays are diagnostic, and surgical treatment pins the femoral head back in place.

Septic hip is another orthopedic emergency. It is seen in little toddlers who have had a febrile illness and then refuse to move the hip. They hold the leg with the hip flexed, in slight abduction and external rotation, and do not let anybody try to move it passively. They have elevated sedimentation rate. Diagnosis is made by aspiration of the hip under general anesthesia, and further open drainage is done if pus is obtained.

Other Locations

Acute hematogenous osteomyelitis is also seen in little kids who have had a febrile illness, but it shows up with severe localized pain in a bone (and no history of trauma to that bone). X-rays will not show anything for a couple of weeks. MRI gives prompt diagnosis. Treat with antibiotics.

Genu varum (bowlegs) is normal up to the age of 3. No treatment is needed. Persistent varus beyond age 3 is most commonly Blount disease (a disturbance of the medial proximal tibial growth plate), for which surgery can be done.

Genu valgus (knock-knee) is normal between ages 4 and 8. No treatment is needed.

Osgood-Schlatter disease (osteochondrosis of the tibial tubercle) is seen in teenagers with persistent pain right over the tibial tubercle, which is aggravated by contraction of the quadriceps. Physical exam shows localized pain right over the tibial tubercle, and there is no knee swelling. First responders use conservative management, as suggested by the mnemonic RICE: rest, ice, compression, and elevation. If such measures are unsuccessful, these patients are referred to an orthopedic surgeon, who at most would use an extension or cylinder cast for 4 to 6 weeks.

Club foot (talipes equinovarus) is seen at birth. Both feet are turned inward, and there is plantar flexion of the ankle, inversion of the foot, adduction of the forefoot, and internal rotation of the tibia. Serial plaster casts started in the neonatal period provide sequential correction starting with the adducted forefoot, then the hindfoot varus, and last the equinus. Often Achilles tenotomy and part-time, long-term use of braces are added. Those who do not respond to casting require surgery, typically done between the ages of 9 and 12 months.

Scoliosis is seen primarily in adolescent girls, whose thoracic spines are curved toward the right. The most sensitive screening finding is to look at the girl from behind while she bends forward, a hump will be noted over her right thorax. The deformity progresses until skeletal maturity is reached (at the onset of menses skeletal maturity is about 80%). In addition to the cosmetic deformity, severe cases develop decreased pulmonary function. Bracing is used to arrest progression; severe cases may need surgery.

Fractures

Remodeling occurs to an astonishing degree in children's fractures, thus degrees of angulation that would be unacceptable in the adult may be okay when these fractures are reduced and immobilized. Also, the healing process is much faster than in the adult. The only areas where children have special problems include supracondylar fractures of the humerus and fractures of any bone that involve the growth plate.

Supracondylar fractures of the humerus occur with hyperextension of the elbow in a child who falls on the hand, with the arm extended. Vascular or nerve injuries can easily occur, and they could lead to Volkmann contracture. Although they can be treated with the appropriate casting or traction (and seldom need surgery), they require careful monitoring of vascular and nerve integrity, and vigilance regarding development of a compartment syndrome.

Fractures that involve the growth plate can be treated by closed reduction if the epiphyses and growth plate are displaced laterally from the metaphysis but are in one piece (i.e., the fracture does not cross the epiphyses or growth plate and does not involve the joint). If the growth plate is in 2 pieces, the very precise alignment provided by open reduction and internal fixation will be required. Otherwise, growth will occur unevenly, resulting in deformity of the extremity.

Tumors

Children and Young Adults

Primary malignant bone tumors are diseases of young people. They complain of persistent low-grade pain, present for several months. The x-ray appearance includes invasion of the adjacent soft tissues, a "sunburst" pattern, and periosteal "onion skinning." Treatment is highly specialized, best left to the experts.

Osteogenic sarcoma is the most common primary malignant bone tumor. It is seen in ages 10–25, usually around the knee (lower femur or upper tibia). A typical "sunburst" pattern is often described on x-rays.

Ewing sarcoma is the second most common; it affects younger children (5–15), and it grows in the diaphyses of long bones. A typical "onion skinning"–type pattern is often seen on x-rays.

Adults

Most malignant bone tumors in adults are metastatic, from the breast in women (lytic lesions), from prostate in men (blastic lesions). Localized pain is an early finding. X-rays can be diagnostic, CT scans give more information, and MRI is even better. Sometimes lytic lesions show up with pathologic fracture (i.e., fracture precipitated by events that would not justify it, such as lifting a bag of groceries).

Multiple myeloma is seen in old men, with fatigue, anemia, and localized pain at specific places on several bones. X-rays are diagnostic, showing multiple punched-out lytic lesions. They also have Bence-Jones protein in the urine and abnormal immunoglobulins in the blood, best shown by serum immunoelectrophoresis. It is treated with chemotherapy. Thalidomide can be used in the event that chemotherapy fails.

Soft tissue sarcomas have relentless growth (several months) of soft tissue mass anywhere in the body. They are firm, fixed to surrounding structures. They metastasize to lungs but not to lymph nodes. MRIs may help diagnose malignancy (but not specific type). Incisional biopsy should be done by the expert who is going to do the treatment, which includes very wide local excision, radiation, and chemotherapy.

General Orthopedics

Common Adult Orthopedic Injuries

X-rays for suspected fractures should always include two views at 90° to one another and always include the joints above and below the broken bone. If the mechanism of injury suggests it, other x-rays should be taken of the bones that are "in the line of force," which might also be broken (for instance, the lumbar spine when somebody falls from a height and lands on—and breaks—his feet).

As a general rule, broken bones that are not badly displaced or angulated or that can be satisfactorily aligned by external manipulation can be immobilized in a cast ("closed reduction"). Broken bones that are severely displaced or angulated or that cannot be aligned easily require surgical intervention to reduce and fix the fracture ("open reduction and internal fixation").

Clavicular fractures are typically at the junction of middle and distal thirds. The traditional treatment is a figure-of-eight device that, by pulling back on both shoulders, aligns the bone. Wearing a sling is more comfortable and also works well. If very precise outcome is desired for cosmetic reasons, open reduction and internal fixation can be done.

Anterior dislocation of the shoulder is by far the most common shoulder dislocation. Patients hold the arm close to their body but rotated outward as if they were going to shake hands. There may be numbness in a small area over the deltoid, from stretching of the axillary nerve. AP and lateral x-rays are diagnostic. Some patients develop recurrent dislocations with minimal trauma.

Posterior shoulder dislocation is rare and occurs after massive uncoordinated muscle contractions, such as epileptic seizure or electrical burn. The arm is held in the usual protective position (close to the body, internally rotated). Regular x-rays can easily miss it; axillary views or scapular lateral views are needed.

Colles fracture results from fall on an outstretched hand, often in old osteoporotic women. The deformed and painful wrist looks like a "dinner fork." The main lesion is a dorsally displaced, dorsally angulated fracture of the distal radius. Treat with close reduction and long arm cast.

Monteggia fracture results from direct blow to the ulna (such as on a raised protective arm hit by a nightstick). There is diaphyseal fracture of the proximal ulna, with anterior dislocation of the radial head.

Galeazzi fracture is the mirror image of the previous one: the distal third of the radius gets the direct blow and has the fracture, and there is dorsal dislocation of the distal radioulnar joint. In both of these, the broken bone often requires open reduction and internal fixation, whereas the dislocated one is typically handled with closed reduction.

Fracture of the scaphoid (carpal navicular) affects a young adult who falls on an outstretched hand. Patient complains of wrist pain. Physical exam shows localized tenderness to palpation over the anatomic snuffbox. In undisplaced fractures, x-rays are usually negative, but thumb spica cast is indicated just with the history and physical findings. X-rays will show the fracture 3 weeks later. If original x-rays show displaced and angulated fracture, open reduction and internal fixation are needed. Scaphoid fractures are notorious for a very high rate of nonunion.

Metacarpal neck fractures (typically the fourth or fifth, or both) happen when a closed fist hits a hard surface (like a wall). The hand is swollen and tender, and x-rays are diagnostic. Treatment depends on the degree of angulation, displacement, or rotary malalignment: closed reduction and ulnar gutter splint for the mild ones; Kirschner wire or plate fixation for the bad ones.

Hip fractures typically happen to the old who sustain a fall. The hip hurts, and the patient's position in the stretcher is classic: The affected leg is shortened and externally rotated. Specific treatment depends on specific location (as shown by x-rays).

Femoral neck fractures, particularly if displaced, compromise the very tenuous blood supply of the femoral head. Faster healing and earlier mobilization can be achieved by replacing the femoral head with a prosthesis.

Intertrochanteric fractures are less likely to lead to avascular necrosis and are usually treated with open reduction and internal fixation. The unavoidable immobilization that ensues poses a very high risk for deep venous thrombosis and pulmonary emboli, thus post-op anticoagulation is recommended.

Femoral shaft fractures are often treated with intramedullary rod fixation. If bilateral and comminuted, they may produce enough internal blood loss to lead to shock (external fixation may help while the patient is stabilized). If they are open, they are an orthopedic emergency, requiring OR cleaning and closure within 6 hours. If multiple, they may lead to the fat embolism syndrome.

Knee injuries typically produce swelling of the knee (knee pain without swelling is unlikely to be a serious knee injury). Swelling of the knee has been described as "the poor man's MRI," a reference to its clinical reliability, and to the fact that MRI is the best highly technological way to look inside the knee.

Collateral ligament injuries are usually sustained in a sideways blow to the knee (a common sports injury). Medial blows disrupt the lateral ligaments, and vice versa. The knee will be swollen and show localized pain by direct palpation on the affected side. With the knee flexed 30°, passive abduction or adduction will produce pain on the torn ligaments and allow further displacement than the normal leg. Abduction demonstrates the medial injuries (valgus stress test), whereas adduction diagnoses the lateral injuries (varus stress test). Isolated injuries are treated with a hinged cast. When several ligaments are torn, surgical repair is preferred.

Anterior cruciate ligament injuries are more common than posterior ones. There is severe knee swelling and pain. With the knee flexed 90°, the leg can be pulled anteriorly, like a drawer being opened (anterior drawer test). A similar finding can be elicited with the knee flexed at 20° by grasping the thigh with one hand, and pulling the leg with the other (Lachman test). Posterior cruciate ligament injuries produce the opposite findings. MRIs are diagnostic. Sedentary patients may be treated with immobilization and rehabilitation, whereas athletes require surgical reconstruction. Almost all cruciate injuries are sports-related and require surgery.

Meniscal tears are difficult to diagnose clinically and on x-rays, but are beautifully shown on MRI. Patients often have protracted pain and swelling after a knee injury, and they may describe catching and locking that limit knee motion, and a "click" when the knee is forcefully extended. Repair is done, trying to save as much meniscus as possible.

Complete meniscectomy leads to late development of degenerative arthritis.

Injuries to the medial meniscus, the medial collateral, and the anterior cruciate often occur simultaneously.

Tibial stress fractures are seen in young men subjected to forced marches. There is tenderness to palpation over a very specific point on the bone, but x-rays are initially normal. Treat with a cast and repeat the x-rays in 2 weeks. Non–weight bearing (crutches) is another option.

Leg fractures involving the tibia and fibula are often seen when a pedestrian is hit by a car. Physical exam shows angulation; x-rays are diagnostic. Casting takes care of the ones that are easily reduced; intramedullary nailing is needed for the ones that cannot be aligned. The lower leg (along with the forearm) is one of the most common locations for development of the compartment syndrome. Increasing pain after a long leg cast has been applied requires immediate removal of the cast and appropriate assessment.

Rupture of the Achilles tendon is seen in out-of-shape middle-aged men who subject themselves to severe strain (tennis, for instance). As they plant the foot and change direction, a loud popping noise is heard (like a rifle shot), and they fall clutching the ankle. Limited plantarflexion is still possible; but pain, swelling, and limping bring them to the doctor. Palpation of the tendon reveals a gap. Casting in equinus position allows healing in several months; surgery achieves quicker cure.

Fractures of the ankle occur when falling on an inverted or everted foot. In either case, both malleoli break. AP, lateral, and mortise x-rays are diagnostic. Open reduction and internal fixation is needed if the fragments are displaced.

Orthopedic Emergencies

The **compartment syndrome** occurs most frequently in the forearm or lower leg. Precipitating events include prolonged ischemia followed by reperfusion, crushing injuries, or other types of trauma. In the lower leg, by far the most common cause is a fracture with closed reduction. The patient has pain and limited use of the extremity. The compartment feels very tight and tender to palpation. The most reliable physical finding is excruciating pain with passive extension. Pulses may be normal. Emergency fasciotomy is required for treatment.

Pain under a cast is always handled by removing the cast and examining the limb.

Open fractures (the broken bone sticking out through a wound) require cleaning in the OR and suitable reduction within 6 hours from the time of the injury.

Posterior dislocation of the hip occurs when the femur is driven backward, such as in a head-on car collision where the knees hit the dashboard. The patient has hip pain and lies in the stretcher with the leg shortened, adducted, and internally rotated (in a broken hip the leg is also shortened, but it is externally rotated). Because of the tenuous blood supply of the femoral head, emergency reduction is needed to avoid avascular necrosis.

Gas gangrene occurs with deep, penetrating, dirty wounds (stepping on a rusty nail, with lots of mud or manure). In about 3 days the patient is extremely sick, looking toxic and moribund. The affected site is tender, swollen, discolored, and has gas crepitation. Treatment includes penicillin and clindamycin, extensive emergency surgical debridement, and hyperbaric oxygen.

Other galloping soft tissue infections are seen primarily in immunocompromised patients (diabetics, AIDS patients), the most common being synergistic bacterial gangrene and necrotizing fasciitis. Patients debilitated by extensive burns or widespread trauma may suffer fulminating fungal infections. The most feared of these is mucormycosis, in which the affected areas turn black; diagnosis is confirmed by tissue biopsy. All of these conditions require repeated, massive surgical excisions of dead tissue in addition to appropriate antibiotics (broad spectrum for synergistic bacterial gangrene and necrotizing fasciitis, IV amphotericin B for mucormycosis).

Associated neurovascular injuries

The radial nerve can be injured in oblique fractures of the middle to distal thirds of the humerus. If the patient comes in unable to dorsiflex (extend) the wrist and regains function when the fracture is reduced and the arm is placed on a hanging cast or coaptation sling, no surgical exploration is needed. However, if nerve paralysis develops or remains after reduction, the nerve is entrapped and surgery has to be done.

Popliteal artery injuries can occur in posterior dislocations of the knee. Attention to the integrity of pulses, Doppler studies, or CT angio, are key issues. Prompt reduction will minimize vascular compromise. Delayed restoration of flow requires prophylactic fasciotomy.

Injury patterns—the second, hidden fracture

The direction of force that produces an obvious injury may produce another one that is less obvious and needs to be sought.

Falls from a height landing on the feet may have obvious foot or leg fractures. Fractures of the lumbar or thoracic spine may be less obvious, and must be looked for.

Head-on automobile collisions may produce obvious injuries in the face, head, and torso; but if the knees hit the dashboard the femoral heads may be driven backward into the pelvis or out of the acetabulum.

Facial fractures and closed head injuries should always prompt evaluation of the cervical spine.

Common Hand Problems

Carpal tunnel syndrome occurs mostly in women who do repetitive hand work (such as typing). They complain about numbness and tingling in their hands, particularly at night, and in the distribution of the median nerve (radial $3\frac{1}{2}$ fingers). The symptoms can be reproduced by hanging the hand limply for a few minutes, or by tapping, percussing or pressing the median nerve over the carpal tunnel. Initial treatment is splints and anti-inflammatory agents. If unsuccessful, electro-diagnostic studies of nerve conduction are done to justify the need for surgery. Endoscopic release is the currently favored operation.

Trigger finger also favors women. Patients wake up in the middle of the night with a finger acutely flexed, and they are unable to extend it unless they pull it with the other hand. When they do so, there is a painful "snap." Steroid injection is the first line of therapy; surgery is the treatment of last resort.

De Quervain tenosynovitis is seen in young mothers who, as they carry their baby, force their hand into wrist flexion and thumb extension to hold the baby's head. They complain of pain along the radial side of the wrist and the first dorsal compartment. On physical exam the pain can be reproduced by asking her to hold her thumb inside her closed fist, then forcing the wrist into ulnar deviation. Splint and antiinflammatory agents can help, but steroid injection is best. Surgery is rarely needed.

Dupuytren contracture occurs in older men of Norwegian ancestry. There is contracture of the palm of the hand, and palmar fascial nodules can be felt. Steroids or collagenase injections can be helpful. If not, surgery may be needed when the hand can no longer be placed flat on a table.

Felon is an abscess in the pulp of a fingertip, caused by a neglected penetrating injury. Patients complain of throbbing pain and have all the classic findings of an abscess, including fever. Because the pulp is a closed space with multiple fascial trabecula, pressure can build up and lead to tissue necrosis; thus surgical drainage must be urgently done.

Gamekeeper thumb is an injury of the ulnar collateral ligament sustained by forced hyperextension of the thumb (historically suffered by gamekeepers when they killed rabbits by dislocating their necks with a violent blow with the extended thumb—nowadays seen as a skiing injury when the thumb gets stuck in the snow or the ski strap during a fall). On physical exam there is collateral laxity at the thumb-metacarpophalangeal joint, and if untreated it can be dysfunctional and painful, and lead to arthritis. Casting is usually done.

Jersey finger is an injury to the flexor tendon sustained when the flexed finger is forcefully extended (as in someone unsuccessfully grabbing a running person by the jersey). When making a fist, the distal phalanx of the injured finger does not flex with the others.

Mallet finger is the reverse of the previous one. The extended finger is forcefully flexed (a common volleyball injury), and the extensor tendon is ruptured. The tip of the affected finger remains flexed when the hand is extended, resembling a mallet. For both of these injuries, splinting is usually the first line of treatment.

Traumatically amputated digits are surgically reattached whenever possible. The amputated digit should be cleaned with sterile saline, wrapped in a saline-moistened gauze, placed in a sealed plastic bag, and the bag placed on a bed of ice. The digit should not be placed in antiseptic solutions or alcohol, should not be put on dry ice, and should not be allowed to freeze. With the use of electric nerve stimulation to preserve muscular function, entire amputated extremities can be reattached.

Back Pain

Lumbar disk herniation occurs almost exclusively at L4–L5 or L5–S1. The peak age incidence is 45–46. Patients often describe several months of vague aching pain (the "discogenic pain" produced by pressure on the anterior spinal ligament) before they have the sudden onset of the "neurogenic pain" precipitated by an event like attempting to lift a heavy object. The latter is extremely severe, "like an electrical shock that shoots down the leg" (exiting on the side of the big toe in L4–L5, or the side of the little toe in L5–S1), and it is exacerbated by coughing, sneezing, or defecating (if the pain is not exacerbated by those activities, the problem is not a herniated disk). Patients cannot ambulate, and they hold the affected leg flexed. Straight leg-raising test gives excruciating pain. MRI confirms the diagnosis. Spontaneous resolution is the rule, as the body reabsorbs the extruded disc. This process used to be very inconvenient for the patient, requiring 3 weeks of strict bed rest. The advent of pain control specialists, who perform nerve blocks under radiological guidance, has made the recovery period much easier. Surgical intervention is needed if neurologic deficits are progressing (progressive muscle weakness), and emergency intervention is required if there is a cauda equina syndrome.

The cauda equina syndrome (distended bladder, flaccid rectal sphincter, perineal saddle anesthesia) is a surgical emergency requiring immediate decompression.

Ankylosing spondylitis is seen in young men in their 30s or early 40s who complain of chronic back pain and morning stiffness. The pain is worse at rest, and improves with activity. Symptoms are progressive, and x-rays eventually show a "bamboo spine." Antiinflammatory agents and physical therapy are used. Many of these patients have the HLA B-27 antigen, which is also associated with uveitis and inflammatory bowel disease.

Metastatic malignancy should be suspected in the elderly who have progressive back pain that is worse at night and unrelieved by rest or positional changes. Weight loss is often an additional finding. If advanced, x-rays will show the lesions (in women, lytic breast cancer metastases at the pedicles; in men, blastic metastases are from the prostate). At a higher cost, MRI is the best diagnostic tool.

Leg Ulcers

Diabetic ulcers are typically indolent and located at pressure points (heel, metatarsal head, tip of toes). They start because of the neuropathy, and they fail to heal because of the microvascular disease. Theoretically they can be healed with good control of the diabetes and by keeping them clean with the leg elevated for many weeks or months. In reality they often get worse and lead to amputations.

Ulcers from arterial insufficiency are usually as far away from the heart as they can be: at the tip of the toes. They look dirty, with a pale base devoid of granulation tissue. The patient has other manifestations of arteriosclerotic occlusive disease (absent pulses, trophic changes, claudication or rest pain). Workup begins with Doppler studies looking for a pressure gradient (if there isn't one, there is microvascular disease not amenable to surgical therapy). Then CT angio, MRI angio or arteriograms, and surgical revascularization or angioplasty and stents.

In the evaluation of chronic foot ulcers, a workup is often done for both diabetes and arteriosclerotic occlusive disease, inasmuch as both problems often coexist in the same patient.

Venous stasis ulcers develop in chronically edematous, indurated, and hyperpigmented skin above the medial malleolus. The ulcer is painless, with granulating bed. The patient has varicose veins and suffers from frequent bouts of cellulitis. Duplex scan is useful in the workup. Treatment revolves around physical support to keep the veins empty, best done with support stockings measured to fit the patient. Surgery may be required (vein stripping, grafting of the ulcer); endovascular ablation with laser or radiofrequency may also be used.

Marjolin ulcer is a squamous cell carcinoma of the skin developing in a chronic leg ulcer. The classic setting is one of many years of healing and breaking down, such as seen in untreated third-degree burns that underwent spontaneous healing, or in chronic draining sinuses secondary to osteomyelitis. A dirty-looking, deeper ulcer develops at the site, with heaped up tissue growth around the edges. Biopsy is diagnostic. Wide local excision and skin grafting are done.

Foot Pain

Plantar fasciitis is a very common but poorly understood problem affecting older, overweight patients who complain of disabling, sharp heel pain every time their foot strikes the ground. The pain is worse in the mornings. X-rays show a bony spur matching the location of the pain, and physical exam shows exquisite tenderness to palpation over the spur. Yet the bony spur is not the cause of the problem (many asymptomatic people have similar spurs). Spontaneous resolution can be expected in 12–18 months, during which time symptomatic treatment is offered, and removal of the bony spur may help.

Morton neuroma is an inflammation of the common digital nerve at the third interspace, between the third and fourth toes. The neuroma is palpable as a very tender spot there. The cause is typically the use of pointed, high-heeled shoes (or pointed cowboy boots) that force the toes to be bunched together. Conservative management includes analgesics and more sensible shoes, but, if needed, surgical excision can be done.

Gout produces the typical swelling, redness, and exquisite pain of sudden onset at the first metatarsal-phalangeal joint, in a middle-age obese man with high serum uric acid. Uric acid crystals are identified in fluid from the joint. Treatment for the acute attack is done with indomethacin and colchicine. Allopurinol and probenicid are used for chronic control.

CHAPTER 3

Pre-Op and Post-Op Care

Cardiac Risk

Ejection fraction under 35% (normal is 55%) poses prohibitive cardiac risk for noncardiac operations. Incidence of perioperative MI is very high, and mortality for such an event is between 55 and 90%.

Goldman's index of cardiac risk, which dates from 1977, is no longer the preferred method of assessing cardiac risk. Functional status, based on the ability to cope with life's demands, is more commonly used now. But Goldman's remains useful for listing all the findings that predict trouble. They are (in descending order of importance): jugular venous distension, recent myocardial infarction, premature ventricular contractions or any rhythm other than sinus, age over 70, emergency surgery, aortic valvular stenosis, poor medical condition, and surgery within the chest or abdomen. The examination will give particular attention to the high-risk situations that intervention can improve.

Jugular venous distention, which indicates the presence of congestive heart failure, is the worst single finding predicting high cardiac risk. If at all possible, treatment with ACE inhibitors, beta-blockers, digitalis, and diuretics should precede surgery.

Recent transmural or subendocardial MI is the next worst predictor of cardiac complications. Operative mortality within 3 months of the infarct is 40%, but it drops to 6% after 6 months. Thus deferring surgery until then is the best course of action. If surgery is imperative sooner, admission to the intensive care unit (ICU) the day before is recommended to "optimize cardiac variables."

Pulmonary Risk

Smoking is by far the most common cause of increased pulmonary risk, and the problem is compromised ventilation (high PCO_2, low forced expiratory volume in 1 second [FEV_1]), rather than compromised oxygenation. The smoking history, or the presence of chronic obstructive pulmonary disease (COPD) should lead to evaluation. Start with FEV_1, and if it is abnormal, follow with blood gases. Cessation of smoking for 8 weeks and intensive respiratory therapy (physical therapy, expectorants, incentive spirometry, humidified air) should precede surgery.

Hepatic Risk

Two clinical findings and three laboratory values are used to predict **operative mortality** in patients with liver disease: encephalopathy, ascites, serum albumin, prothrombin time (INR), and bilirubin (only as it reflects hepatocyte function). The presence and severity of these factors can be combined in a variety of ways; the current favorite system is Child class, in which class A has 10% mortality, class B 30%, and class C 80%. But specific numbers are misleading, because so many other factors influence the outcome. Suffice it to say that a patient in coma with huge ascites, albumin below 2, INR twice normal, and bilirubin above 4 could not survive a haircut, much less an operation.

Nutritional Risk

Severe nutritional depletion is identified by loss of 20% of body weight over a couple of months, serum albumin below 3, anergy to skin antigens, or serum transferrin level of less than 200 mg/dL (or a combination of the above). Operative risk is multiplied manyfold in those circumstances. Surprisingly, as few as 4 or 5 days of pre-operative nutritional support (preferably via the gut) can make a big difference, and 7–10 days would be optimal if the surgery can be deferred that long.

Metabolic Risk

Diabetic coma is an absolute contraindication to surgery. Rehydration, return of urinary output, and at least partial correction of the acidosis and hyperglycemia have to be achieved before surgery. (If the indication for surgery is a septic process, complete correction of all variables will be impossible as long as the septic process is present.)

Postoperative Complications

Fever

Malignant hyperthermia develops shortly after the onset of the anesthetic (halothane or succinylcholine). Temperature exceeds 104°F. Metabolic acidosis and hypercalcemia also occur. A family history may exist. Treat with IV dantrolene, 100% oxygen, correction of the acidosis, and cooling blankets. Watch for development of myoglobinuria.

Bacteremia is seen within 30–45 minutes of invasive procedures (instrumentation of the urinary tract is a classic example), and there are chills and temperature spike to or exceeding 104°F. Do blood cultures times three, start empiric antibiotics.

Although rare, severe wound pain and very high fever within hours of surgery should alert you to the possibility of gas gangrene in the surgical wound.

Postoperative (PO) fever in the usual range (101°–103°F) is caused (sequentially in time) by atelectasis, pneumonia, urinary tract infection, deep venous thrombophlebitis, wound infection, or deep abscesses.

Atelectasis is the most common source of post-op fever on the first PO day. Rule out the other causes listed above, listen to the lungs, do chest x-ray, improve ventilation (deep breathing and coughing, postural drainage, incentive spirometry). The ultimate therapy if needed is bronchoscopy.

Pneumonia will happen in about 3 days if atelectasis is not resolved. Fever will persist. Chest x-ray will show infiltrates. Do sputum cultures, treat with appropriate antibiotics.

Urinary tract infection typically produces fever starting on PO day 3. Work up with urinalysis, urinary cultures. Treat with appropriate antibiotics.

Deep thrombophlebitis typically produces fever starting on PO day 5 or thereabouts. Doppler studies of deep leg and pelvic veins is the best diagnostic modality (physical exam is worthless). Anticoagulate with heparin, transitioning later to warfarin.

Wound infection typically begins to produce fever on PO day 7. Physical exam will show erythema, warmth, and tenderness. Treat with antibiotics if there is only cellulitis; open and drain the wound if an abscess is present. When these two cannot be easily distinguished clinically, sonogram is diagnostic.

Deep abscesses (like subphrenic, pelvic, or subhepatic) start producing fever around PO days 10–15. CT scan of the appropriate body cavity is diagnostic. Percutaneous radiologically guided drainage is therapeutic.

Chest Pain

Perioperative myocardial infarction may occur during the operation (triggered most commonly by hypotension), in which case it is detected by the EKG monitor (ST depression, T-wave flattening). When it happens post-op, it is typically within the first 2–3 post-op days, showing up as chest pain only in one-third of the cases, and with the complications of the MI in the rest. The most reliable diagnostic test is troponin. Mortality (50–90%) greatly exceeds that of MI not associated with surgery. Treatment is directed at the complications. Clot busters cannot be used in the perioperative setting, but emergency angioplasty and coronary stent may be used.

Pulmonary embolus (PE) typically happens around PO day 7 in elderly and/or immobilized patients. The pain is pleuritic, of sudden onset, and is accompanied by shortness of breath. The patient is anxious, diaphoretic, and tachycardic, with prominent distended veins in the neck and forehead (a low CVP virtually excludes the diagnosis). Arterial blood gases show hypoxemia and hypocapnia. The standard diagnostic test is a spiral CT with intravenous dye, commonly referred to as a CT angio. After confirming the diagnosis, start treatment with heparinization. Add an inferior vena cava filter (Greenfield) if PEs recur during anticoagulation or if anticoagulation is contraindicated.

Prevention of thromboembolism will in turn prevent PE. Sequential compression devices can be used on anyone who does not have a lower extremity fracture. In high risk patients, anticoagulation is indicated. Risk factors include age >40, pelvic or leg fractures, venous injury, femoral venous catheter, and anticipated prolonged immobilization.

Other Pulmonary Complications

Aspiration is a distinct hazard in awake intubations in combative patients with a full stomach. It can be lethal right away, or lead to chemical injury of the tracheobronchial tree and subsequent pulmonary failure, or secondary pneumonia. Prevention includes NPO and antacids before induction. Therapy starts with lavage and removal of acid and particulate matter (with the help of bronchoscopy), followed by bronchodilators and respiratory support.

Intraoperative tension pneumothorax can develop in patients with traumatized lungs (recent blunt trauma with punctures by broken ribs) once they are subjected to positive-pressure breathing. They become progressively more difficult to "bag," BP steadily declines and

CVP steadily rises. If the abdomen is open, quick decompression can be achieved through the diaphragm. If not, a needle can be inserted through the anterior chest wall into the pleural space (sneaking in under the drapes). Formal chest tube has to be placed later.

Disorientation/Coma

Hypoxia is the first thing that has to be suspected when a post-op patient gets confused and disoriented. It may be secondary to sepsis. Check blood gases, provide respiratory support.

Adult respiratory distress syndrome (ARDS) is seen in patients with a stormy, complicated post-op course, often complicated by sepsis as the precipitating event. There are bilateral pulmonary infiltrates and hypoxia, with no evidence of congestive heart failure. The centerpiece of therapy is positive end-expiratory pressure (PEEP), taking care not to use excessive volume. Excessive ventilatory volumes have been shown to result in baro-trauma. A source of sepsis must be sought and corrected. There is mounting evidence that extracorporeal membrane oxygenation (ECMO) is becoming the new standard of care for ARDS refractory to PEEP. The main complication is intracranial bleeding, which can be minimized by using a venovenous connection to hook up the patient to the machine.

Delirium tremens (DTs) is very common in the alcoholic whose drinking is suddenly interrupted by surgery. About the second or third PO day they get confused, have hallucinations, and become combative. Intravenous benzodiazepines are the standard therapy, but alcohol is also effective. It can be intravenous (5% alcohol in 5% dextrose), or for those on oral intake we can actually prescribe their favorite drink.

Hyponatremia, if quickly induced by liberal administration of sodium-free IV fluids (like D5W) in a postoperative patient with high levels of antidiuretic hormone (ADH; triggered by the response to trauma), will produce confusion, convulsions, and eventually coma and often death ("water intoxication"). Chart review confirms large fluid intake, quick weight gain, and rapidly lowering serum sodium concentration (in a matter of hours). The problem is best prevented by including sodium in the IV fluids. Once it happens, therapy is controversial and mortality is very high (young women are particularly vulnerable). Most authors use small amounts of hypertonic saline (aliquots of 100 mL of 5%, or 500 mL of 3%), perhaps add osmotic diuretics.

Hypernatremia can also be a source of confusion, lethargy, and potentially coma—if rapidly induced by large, unreplaced water loss. Surgical damage to the posterior pituitary with unrecognized diabetes insipidus is a good example. Unrecognized osmotic diuresis can also do it. Chart review will show large, unreplaced urinary output, rapid weight loss, and rapidly rising serum sodium concentration. Rapid replacement of the fluid deficit is needed, but to "cushion" the impact on tonicity many prefer to use D5$\frac{1}{2}$ or D5$\frac{1}{3}$ normal saline (NS), rather than D5W.

Ammonium intoxication is a common source of coma in the cirrhotic patient with bleeding esophageal varices who undergoes a portocaval shunt.

Urinary Complications

Postoperative urinary retention is extremely common, particularly after surgery in the lower abdomen, pelvis, perineum, or groin. The patient feels the need to void, but cannot do it. In-and-out bladder catheterization should be done at 6 hours post-op if no spontaneous voiding has occurred. Indwelling (Foley) catheter is indicated at the second (some say third) consecutive catheterization.

Zero urinary output typically is caused by a mechanical problem, rather than a biologic one. Look for plugged or kinked catheter.

Low urinary output (less than 0.5 mL/kg/h) in the presence of normal perfusing pressure (i.e., not because of shock) represents either fluid deficit or acute renal failure. A low-tech diagnostic test is a fluid challenge: a bolus of 500 mL of IV fluid infused over

10 or 20 minutes. Dehydrated patients will respond with a temporary increase in urinary output, those in renal failure will not do so. A more elegant way to decide is to measure urinary sodium: it will be less than 10 or 20 mEq/L in the dehydrated patient with good kidneys, while it will exceed 40 mEq/L in cases of renal failure. An even more sophisticated way to express the same is to determine "fractional excretion of sodium," which in renal failure exceeds 1.

Abdominal Distention

Paralytic ileus is to be expected in the first few days after abdominal surgery. Bowel sounds are absent, there is no passage of gas. There may be mild distension, but there is no pain. Paralytic ileus is prolonged by hypokalemia.

Early mechanical bowel obstruction because of adhesions can happen during the postoperative period. What was probably assumed to be paralytic ileus not resolving after 5, 6, or 7 days is most likely an early mechanical bowel obstruction. X-rays will show dilated loops of small bowel and air-fluid levels. Diagnosis is confirmed with an abdominal CT scan that demonstrates a transition point between proximal dilated bowel and distal collapsed bowel at the site of the obstruction. Surgical intervention is needed to correct the problem.

Ogilvie syndrome is a poorly understood (but very common) condition that could be described as a "paralytic ileus of the colon." It does not follow abdominal surgery, but classically is seen in elderly sedentary patients (Alzheimer, nursing home) who have become further immobilized owing to surgery elsewhere (broken hip, prostatic surgery). They develop large abdominal distention (tense but not tender), and imaging studies show a massively dilated colon. After fluid and electrolyte correction, the safest thing to do is perform a colonoscopy, suck out all the air, and place a long rectal tube. IV neostigmine stimulates colonic motility, but this drug is best avoided. It has lots of side effects and is lethal if inadvertently given to someone whose colon is actually obstructed.

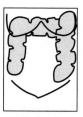

Radiological appearance of dilated colon

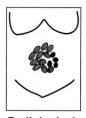

Radiological appearance of dilated small bowel

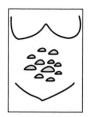

Air fluid levels described in the following box

Is It Small Bowel or Colon?

If you look at vertical sections of a CT scan of the abdomen that shows dilated bowel, how can you tell if you are looking at small bowel or colon? There are 3 clues:

1. *Location.* The colon hugs the outside boundaries of the image, while the small bowel tends to be in the center of it.

2. *Size* is very, very helpful. Make a circle between your index finger and thumb, and hold it right in front of your face: That is about as big as small bowel can get. Now make a circle with both hands, with index touching index, and thumb touching thumb: The colon can attain that size.

3. *Fine details.* The edges of the colon have small indentations (haustral markings), whereas the small bowel has little lines going across ("stacked coins").

What Are Air-Fluid Levels?

Everyone has air and fluid in the GI tract. But the churning motion of normal peristalsis makes a foam out of those. If the small bowel is obstructed, it eventually gets tired of trying to push the stuff, so that the liquid goes to the bottom and the air stays at the top. A horizontal line divides these, which can be seen in images taken with the patient in the upright position.

Wound

Wound dehiscence is typically seen around the fifth post-op day after open laparotomy. The wound looks intact, but large amounts of pink, "salmon-colored" fluid are noted to be soaking the dressings (it is peritoneal fluid). The wound has to be taped securely, the abdomen bound, and mobilization and coughing done with great care, while arrangements are made for prompt reoperation to prevent evisceration now or ventral hernia later on.

Evisceration is a catastrophic complication of wound dehiscence, where the skin itself opens up and the abdominal contents rush out. It typically happens when the patient (who may not have been recognized as having a dehiscence) coughs, strains, or gets out of bed. The patient must be kept in bed, and the bowel be covered with large sterile dressings soaked with warm saline. Emergency abdominal closure is required.

Wound infections are typically seen around the seventh post-op day. (They were described under the heading of postoperative fever.)

Fistulas of the GI tract are recognized because bowel contents leak out through a wound or drain site. They may harm the patient in a number of ways. If they do not empty directly and completely to the outside, but leak into a "cesspool" that then leaks out, the problem will be sepsis (requiring complete drainage). If they drain freely (patient is afebrile, with no signs of peritoneal irritation), there are three potential problems: fluid and electrolyte loss, nutritional depletion, and erosion and digestion of the belly wall. These problems are related to location and volume of the fistula: nonexistent in the distal colon, present but manageable in low-volume (up to 200–300 mL/day) high GI fistulas (stomach, duodenum, upper jejunum), and daunting in high-volume (several liters per day) fistulas high in the GI tract. Fluid and electrolyte replacement, nutritional support (preferably elemental diets delivered beyond the fistula), and compulsive protection of the abdominal wall (suction tubes, "ostomy" bags) are done to keep the patient alive until nature heals the fistula. Nature will do so if there is no foreign body, epithelialization, tumor, infection, irradiated tissue, inflammatory bowel disease, or distal obstruction (the "F.E.T.I.D." mnemonic) to prevent it. Steroids will also prevent healing.

Intravenous Fluid Therapy

If surgical patients cannot eat and drink, we have to put them on intravenous fluids. Those always include what we call "maintenance" IV therapy. Sometimes we have to do more, providing "replacement" and/or "correction." Let's consider these IV therapies one at a time.

In principle, "maintenance" is the equivalent of what a patient would have eaten and drunk if they were not sick. In practice, we include only 3 things for a few days: water, sodium, and potassium. Plain water cannot be infused, because it would lyse the red blood cells. To make it isotonic and safe, we typically add dextrose at 5% concentration (the famous "D5W"). A standard adult would receive an infusion of about 2–3 liters of D5W a day—which does double duty, because it also minimizes the protein breakdown of complete starvation.

For sodium and potassium, the amount to remember is around 100 mEq per day of each, but with a twist: Absent congestive heart failure or liver disease, we have enormous flexibility with sodium. It should not be zero and should not exceed a few hundred milliequivalents, but anything between 50 and 250 is fair game; precision is not required. Normal saline has 154 mEq/L of sodium, and 5% dextrose in one-half normal saline is often used as the vehicle for sodium. For potassium, the guiding principle is to link the dose to caloric intake. Total parenteral nutrition would require more than 100 mEq per day of potassium—but for just a few days of semistarvation, 40–60 mEq per day suffices. We typically use ampules of potassium chloride as the source.

(continued)

Intravenous Fluid Therapy (*Cont'd*)

By far the most common maintenance IV fluid order reads: "Dextrose 5 percent in one-half normal saline, with 20 milliequivalents of potassium chloride per liter, to run in at 125 cc per hour." But if you are too lazy to spell all that, the nurses will understand "D5½ NS with 20 mEq of KCl/L, to run in at 125 cc/hr."

Let's move to "replacement." Here we are talking about abnormal fluid losses that have been measured and require infusion, cc per cc, of an appropriate fluid. The most common such losses are from the GI tract: vomiting, nasogastric tube output, fistulas, massive diarrhea, malfunctioning ileostomies, and so on. If the aggregate loss is a small fraction of a patient's basic, maintenance volume, we can replace today what was recorded yesterday, then provide tomorrow what we measured today, and so on. But if the abnormal losses approach or exceed *half of daily basic needs*, more frequent replacement is prudent: every 8 hours, or even every 4.

The composition of the replacement fluid should mimic what was lost. For instance, GI fluids are isotonic with plasma and rich in potassium.

- Fluids from beyond the pylorus are alkaline. Ringer's lactate with a little additional KCl (10–20 mEq/L) will do nicely.

- Pure gastric juice is very acidic. Half-normal saline with a little more potassium (20–40 mEq/L) is an appropriate replacement.

Either fluid should include 5% dextrose: A little extra sugar always helps.

If maintenance and replacement fluids are properly managed from day one, there will be no need for "correction." But if not, the patient will develop a "fluid and electrolyte disorder" that we will have to fix. The paragraphs that follow provide a few examples of these.

Fluids and Electrolytes

Hypernatremia invariably means that the patient has lost water (or other hypotonic fluids) and has developed hypertonicity. Every 3 mEq/L that the serum sodium concentration is above 140 represents roughly 1 L of water lost. If the problem happens slowly (several days), the brain will adapt, and the only clinical manifestations will be those of volume depletion. Therapy requires volume repletion, but it must be done so that the volume is corrected rapidly (in a matter of hours), while the tonicity is only gently "nudged" in the right direction (and goes back to normal in a matter of days). This is achieved by using D5$\frac{1}{2}$ NS rather than D5W. Hypernatremia of rapid development (such as in osmotic diuresis or diabetes insipidus) will produce CNS symptoms (the brain has not had time to adapt), and correction can be safely done with more diluted fluid (D5$\frac{1}{3}$ NS, or even D5W).

Hyponatremia means that water has been retained and hypotonicity has developed, but there are two different scenarios (easily distinguishable by the clinical circumstances). In one, a patient who starts with normal fluid volume adds to it by retaining water because of the presence of inappropriate amounts of ADH (for instance, post-op water intoxication, or inappropriate ADH secreted by tumors). In the other, a patient who is losing large amounts of isotonic fluids (typically from the GI tract) is forced to retain water if he has not received appropriate replacement with isotonic fluids. Rapidly developing hyponatremia (water intoxication) produces CNS symptoms (the brain has not had time to adapt), and requires careful use of hypertonic saline (3% or 5%). In slowly developing hyponatremia from inappropriate ADH, the brain has time to adapt, and therapy should be water restriction. In the case of the hypovolemic, dehydrated patient losing GI fluids and forced to retain water, volume restoration with isotonic fluids (NS or Ringer lactate) will provide prompt correction of the hypovolemia and allow the body to slowly and safely unload the retained water and return the tonicity to normal. The choice between the two is determined by acid-base status. Use normal saline only if there is alkalosis. Ringer lactate is better for acidotic patients and those whose pH is normal.

Hypokalemia develops slowly (days) when potassium is lost from the GI tract (all GI fluids have lots of K), or in the urine (because of loop diuretics, or too much aldosterone), and it is not replaced. Hypokalemia develops very rapidly (hours) when potassium moves into the cells, most notably when diabetic ketoacidosis is corrected. Therapy is obviously potassium replacement. Remember that the safe "speed limit" of IV potassium administration is 10 mEq/h (which can be exceeded only if you know what you are doing).

Hyperkalemia will occur slowly if the kidney cannot excrete potassium (renal failure, aldosterone antagonists), and it will occur rapidly if potassium is being dumped from the cells into the blood (crushing injuries, dead tissue, acidosis). The ultimate therapy for hyperkalemia is hemodialysis, but while waiting for it we can help by "pushing potassium into the cells" (50% dextrose and insulin), sucking it out of the GI tract (NG suction, exchange resins), or neutralizing its effect on the cellular membrane (IV calcium). The latter provides the quickest protection.

---

pH or Nanoequivalents?

The pH scale was invented in 1909 by a Danish biochemist by the name of Sorensen. He was not a physician. He dealt with the enormous scale of hydrogen ion concentrations in nature, which range from 1 to 0.000 000 000 000 01. Converting that to a scale from 1 to 14 was no mean feat.

But we medical practitioners do not have to contend with such a vast spectrum in the blood of patients. We should never have adopted the pH scale. It is counterintuitive. First, it is upside-down: More hydrogen ions = lower pH. Second, it is not linear: It's a logarithm. Decimal points in the pH do not convey the true magnitude of H^+ changes in the blood, which can go from 20 to 120.

(continued)

---

pH or Nanoequivalents? (*Cont'd*)

We are comfortable measuring blood electrolytes in milliequivalents. Hydrogen ion is just another electrolyte, albeit one we have in tiny amounts. Moving the decimal point to the right gives us a suitable unit: nanoequivalents. The normal is 40. The minimum concentration compatible with life is 20 (severe alkalosis), and the maximum is 120 (horrible acidosis). Easy to grasp. Intuitive. Linear. Perfect.

But there is more. As you know, acid-base balance has two components, metabolic and respiratory. We measure the latter with pCO_2, and by a happy coincidence the normal happens to be 40. Normal amount of hydrogen ion in the blood: 40 nanoequivalents. Normal partial pressure of CO_2: 40. Those two values are reported by the lab with the blood gases. When you see 40 and 40, you know everything is okay. The other report that comes with the electrolytes will confirm the bicarbonate is also in good shape.

When a patient has a pure respiratory problem, those two numbers we get with the blood gases move pretty much in parallel. If they do not, you are instantly alerted to the fact that there is a metabolic problem as well. Either both systems are deranged, or one is compensating for the other. Your clinical skills—history and physical—then take over and solve the puzzle. Neat.

If this topic bores you, just turn the page and keep using pH. No big deal. If it intrigues you, I suggest you read a little book published by Lippincott, Williams & Wilkins called *Fluids and Electrolytes in the Surgical Patient*. It had five editions in the U.S. and was translated and published in Spanish, Italian, and Greek. I highly recommend it. But I am biased.

I wrote that thing.

Metabolic acidosis can occur from excessive production of fixed acids (diabetic ketoacidosis, lactic acidosis, low-flow states), from loss of buffers (loss of bicarbonate-rich fluids from the GI tract), or from inability of the kidney to eliminate fixed acids (renal failure). In all 3 cases the blood pH is low (<7.4), the serum bicarbonate is low (<25), and there is a base deficit. When abnormal acids are piling up in the blood, there is also an "anion gap" (serum sodium exceeds by more than 10 or 15 the sum of chloride and bicarbonate), which does not exist when the problem is loss of buffers. The treatment in all cases must be directed at the underlying cause. If it is loss of bicarbonate, we should replace bicarbonate or use bicarbonate precursors, such as lactate or acetate.

In all cases of longstanding acidosis, of whichever etiology, renal loss of K^+ leads to a deficit that does not become obvious until the acidosis is corrected. Thus we must be prepared to replace potassium as part of our therapy.

Metabolic alkalosis occurs from loss of acid gastric juice, or from excessive administration of bicarbonate (or precursors). There is a high blood pH (>7.4), high serum bicarbonate (>25), and a base excess. In most cases, an abundant intake of KCl (between 5 to 10 mEq/h) will allow the kidney to correct the problem. Only rarely is ammonium chloride or 0.1 N HCl needed.

Respiratory acidosis or alkalosis results from impaired ventilation (acidosis) or abnormal hyperventilation (alkalosis). They are recognized by abnormal PCO_2 (low in alkalosis, high in acidosis) in conjunction with the abnormal pH of the blood. The therapy must be directed at improving ventilation (in acidosis) or reducing it (in alkalosis).

Radiology for the Surgical Consumer

I am not a radiologist, but as a clinician I use their products. This brief overview of what is available, the indications for each study, and their relative cost will help you determine which way to go in many examination questions.

Plain x-ray. About $20. X-rays are widely available but handicapped by several limitations: They cannot penetrate the skull; they use ionizing radiation; and they superimpose the densities of all the tissues they go through. They can only see black, white, and a few shades of gray. In many applications x-rays have already been superseded by CT scans, but they are still useful where black and white suffice: broken or dislocated bones, and chest x-rays.

Sonogram. About $150. A transmitter aims sound beams at the target, and echoes are read back. The readings are used to create images (sonogram, ultrasound, or echo—different names for the same thing) or to measure flow by using the Doppler principle. If you get both, we call that "duplex" scanning. Sonograms are best at the interface of solid and liquid (perfect for gallstones or urinary tract obstruction, and an echocardiogram is our standard way to look at morphological abnormalities of the heart). The enemy of sonograms is air, which makes the echoes harder to read. Sonograms have many limitations—they cannot go through bones, and they are very much operator dependent, both to conduct and to read. (To nonspecialists, the images look like "black-and-white TV on the blink.") But there is no safer way to look inside a human being: Nothing needs to be injected. There is no radiation. The only way to kill a patient with an ultrasound is to hit him over the head with the sonogram machine.

(continued)

Radiology for the Surgical Consumer (*Cont'd*)

CT scan. About $350. Computed tomography (CT) scans are glorified x-rays. They use the same basic ionizing radiation, but now aimed from many different angles and put together by a computer. They are capable of penetrating the skull and showing black, white, and hundreds of shades of gray. CT scans have taken over for head trauma, the cervical spine, the abdomen, kidney stones, and many other applications where x-rays were used in the past.

MRI. About $1,500. Much more expensive and not as widely available as the CT, magnetic resonance imaging (MRI) gives much more detail. MRI was first known as "magnetic nuclear resonance," which patients rejected outright. (When patients heard the word "nuclear," they thought about atomic bombs. The technology was renamed.) From a consumer perspective, MRI is just a "glorified CT"—although in reality it is a completely different technology. Magnetic pulses line up elements within the nuclei of the cells, producing exquisitely detailed images. MRI is the first choice for looking at soft, mushy targets in the body: spinal cord, brain tumors, the structures inside the knee, herniated discs, soft tissue sarcomas. MRI is not useful to guide interventional studies, however, because any ferrous metal in the vicinity will go flying across the room when the machine is turned on.

PET scan. About $6,500. A positron emission tomography (PET) scan gives a picture of metabolic activity. It was first used by neuroscientists to see what parts of the brain were active when volunteers were happy, or sad, or angry (or horny). Now PET is used primarily in the workup of lung cancer, to determine whether enlarged mediastinal nodes are old scars from back when the patient dug tunnels for a living or metastases rapidly growing.

Chapter 4
General Surgery

Diseases of the Gastrointestinal System

The Upper Gastrointestinal System

The esophagus

Gastroesophageal reflux may produce vague symptoms, difficult to distinguish from other sources of epigastric distress. When the diagnosis is uncertain, pH monitoring is best to establish the presence of reflux and its correlation with the symptoms. In more typical cases, an overweight individual complains of burning retrosternal pain and "heartburn" that is brought about by bending over, wearing tight clothing, or lying flat in bed at night; and relieved by the ingestion of antacids or over-the-counter H_2 blockers. If there is a longstanding history, the concern is the damage that might have been done to the lower esophagus (peptic esophagitis) and the possible development of Barrett esophagus. In that setting, endoscopy and biopsies are the indicated tests.

Surgery for gastroesophageal reflux is appropriate in longstanding symptomatic disease that cannot be controlled by medical means; it is necessary in anyone who has developed complications (ulceration, stenosis); and it is imperative if there are severe dysplastic changes. For the latter, radiofrequency ablation should be added to <u>Nissen fundo</u><u>plication</u>. In all other cases, <u>laparoscopic Nissen fundoplication</u> is the usual procedure. wraps fundus around LES

Motility problems have recognizable clinical patterns, such as crushing pain with swallowing in uncoordinated massive contraction; or the suggestive pattern of dysphagia seen in achalasia, where solids are swallowed with less difficulty than liquids. Manometry studies are used for the definitive diagnosis. Barium swallow is typically done first.

Achalasia is seen more commonly in women. There is dysphagia that is worse for liquids; the patient eventually learns that sitting up straight and waiting allows the weight of the column of liquid to overcome the sphincter. There is occasional regurgitation of undigested food. X-rays show megaesophagus. Manometry is diagnostic. The most appealing current treatment is balloon dilatation done by endoscopy.

Cancer of the esophagus shows the classic progression of dysphagia starting with meat, then other solids, then soft foods, eventually liquids, and finally (in several months) saliva. Significant weight loss is always seen. Squamous cell carcinoma is seen in men with a history of smoking and drinking (blacks have high incidence). Adenocarcinoma is seen in people with long-standing gastroesophageal reflux. Diagnosis for both is established with endoscopy and biopsies, but barium swallow must precede the endoscopy to help prevent inadvertent perforation. CT scan assesses operability, but most cases can only get palliative (rather than curative) surgery.

Mallory-Weiss tear occurs after prolonged, forceful vomiting. Eventually, bright red blood comes up. Endoscopy establishes diagnosis and allows photocoagulation (laser). Tears usually @ stomach & esophagus junction

Boerhaave syndrome also starts with prolonged, forceful vomiting leading to esophageal perforation. There is continuous, severe, wrenching epigastric and low sternal pain of sudden onset, soon followed by fever, leukocytosis, and a very sick-looking patient. Contrast swallow (Gastrografin first, barium if negative) is diagnostic, and emergency surgical repair should follow. Delay in diagnosis and treatment has grave consequences.

Instrumental perforation of the esophagus is by far the most common reason for esophageal perforation. Shortly after completion of endoscopy, symptoms as described above will develop. There may be emphysema in the lower neck (virtually diagnostic in this setting). Contrast studies and prompt repair are imperative.

The stomach

Gastric adenocarcinoma is more common in the elderly. There is anorexia, weight loss, and vague epigastric distress or early satiety, Occasionally hematemesis. Endoscopy and biopsies are diagnostic. CT scan helps assess operability. Surgery is the best therapy.

Gastric lymphoma is nowadays almost as common as gastric adenocarcinoma. Presentation and diagnosis are similar, but treatment is based on chemotherapy or radiotherapy. Surgery is done if perforation is feared as the tumor melts away. Low-grade lymphomatoid transformation (MALTOMA) can be reversed by eradication of *H. pylori*.

Gastrointestinal stromal tumors (GISTs) occur mostly in the stomach. Small tumors with few mitoses (for instance, 1 cm and fewer than 5 mitotic figures) are usually benign. Large tumors with many mitotic figures are malignant. The only curative treatment is complete surgical resection. Care must be taken not to rupture the tumor during surgery, to avoid peritoneal contamination. Inoperable, metastatic, or recurrent tumors can be palliated (but not cured) with imatinib (Gleevec).

The Mid and Lower Gastrointestinal System

Small bowel and appendix

Mechanical intestinal obstruction is typically caused by adhesions in those who have had a prior laparotomy. There is colicky abdominal pain and protracted vomiting, progressive abdominal distention (if it is a low obstruction), and no passage of gas or feces. Early on, high-pitched bowel sounds coincide with the colicky pain (after a few days there is silence). X-rays show distended loops of small bowel, with air-fluid levels. Treatment starts with NPO, NG suction, and IV fluids, hoping for spontaneous resolution, while watching for early signs of strangulation. Surgery is done if conservative management is unsuccessful, within 24 hours in cases of complete obstruction or within a few days in cases of partial obstruction.

Strangulated obstruction (compromised blood supply) starts as described above, but eventually the patient develops fever, leukocytosis, constant pain, signs of peritoneal irritation, and ultimately full-blown peritonitis and sepsis. Emergency surgery is required.

Mechanical intestinal obstruction caused by an incarcerated hernia has the same clinical picture and potential for strangulation as described above, but the physical exam shows the irreducible hernia that used to be reducible. Because we can effectively eliminate the hernia (we cannot effectively eliminate adhesions), all of these undergo surgical repair, but the timing varies: emergently after proper rehydration in those who appear to be strangulated; electively in those who can be reduced manually and have viable bowel.

All abdominal hernias should be electively repaired to avoid the risk of intestinal obstruction and strangulation. Exceptions include umbilical hernias in patients younger than 2–5 years of age (they may close by themselves) and esophageal sliding hiatal hernias (which are not "true" hernias). Hernias that become irreducible need emergency surgery to prevent strangulation. Those that have been irreducible for years need elective repair only.

Carcinoid syndrome is seen in patients with a small bowel carcinoid tumor with liver metastases. The syndrome includes diarrhea, flushing of the face, wheezing, and right-sided heart valvular damage (look for prominent jugular venous pulse). Twenty-four-hour urinary collection for 5-hydroxyindoleacetic acid provides the diagnosis. (Hint: Whenever syndromes produce episodic attacks or spells, the offending agent will be at high concentrations in the blood only at the time of the attack. A blood sample taken afterward will be normal. Thus, a 24-hour urinary collection is more likely to provide the diagnosis.)

The classic picture of acute appendicitis begins with anorexia, followed by vague periumbilical pain that several hours later becomes sharp, severe, constant, and localized to the right lower quadrant of the abdomen. Tenderness, guarding, and rebound are found to the right and below the umbilicus (not elsewhere in the belly). There is modest fever and leukocytosis in the 10,000–15,000 range, with neutrophilia and immature forms. Emergency appendectomy should follow.

Doubtful presentations that could be acute appendicitis include any that do not have all the classic findings described above. CT scan has become the standard diagnostic modality for those cases.

Short bowel syndrome. If for any reason a large portion of the small bowel is lost, two factors determine the fate of that patient: the patient's age and the status of the pylorus and ileocecal valve. A young child with those two structures intact has a good chance of survival. An old person lacking them does not.

The colon

Cancer of the right colon typically shows up with anemia (hypochromic, iron deficiency) in the right age group (elderly), for no good reason. Stools will be 4+ for occult blood. Colonoscopy and biopsies are diagnostic; surgery (right hemicolectomy) is treatment of choice.

Cancer of the left colon typically shows with bloody bowel movements. Blood coats the outside of the stool, there may be constipation, stools may have narrow caliber. Flexible proctosigmoidoscopic exam (45 or 60 cm) and biopsies are usually the first diagnostic study. Before surgery is done, full colonoscopy is needed to rule out synchronous second primary. CT scan helps assess operability and extent. Pre-op chemotherapy and radiation may be needed for large rectal cancers.

Colonic polyps may be premalignant. In descending order of probability for malignant degeneration are familial polyposis (and variants such as Gardner), familial multiple inflammatory polyps, villous adenoma, and adenomatous polyp. Polyps that are not premalignant include juvenile, Peutz-Jeghers, isolated inflammatory, and hyperplastic.

Crohn's disease and chronic ulcerative colitis (CUC) produce severe diarrhea with blood and mucus. The former can happen in multiple GI locations, and thus cannot be cured by surgical resection. Crohn's disease is surgically treated only when there are complications such as bleeding, stricture, or fistulization. CUC can be surgically cured, but we are reluctant to do it because the rectal mucosa has to go, leaving the patient with either a stoma or an ileoanal anastomosis, neither of which is pleasant to have. Clear-cut indications include active disease for more than 20 years (malignant degeneration), severe nutritional depletion, multiple hospitalizations, need for high-dose steroids or immunosuppressants, or development of toxic megacolon (fever, leukocytosis, abdominal pain and tenderness, and massively dilated colon with gas within the wall).

Pseudomembranous enterocolitis is caused by overgrowth of *Clostridium difficile* in patients who have been on antibiotics. Any antibiotic can do it. Clindamycin was the first one described, and, currently, cephalosporins are the most common cause. There is profuse, watery diarrhea, crampy abdominal pain, fever, and leukocytosis. The diagnosis is best made by identifying the toxin in the stool. Stool cultures take too long, and the pseudomembranes are not always seen on endoscopy. The culpable antibiotic should be discontinued, and no antidiarrheals should be used. Metronidazole is the treatment of choice, with vancomycin serving as an alternate. A virulent form of the disease, unresponsive to treatment, with a WBC above 50,000 and serum lactate above 5, requires emergency colectomy.

Fecal enema has been recently reported as a very effective cure for the overgrowth of *Clostridium difficile*. It makes sense that restoring normal bowel flora would help in this situation. Yet, besides the "ick" factor, there are still a lot of unanswered questions. How should the donors be selected? What regulatory agency has jurisdiction? Are randomized studies needed? I don't know the answers, but if I had this disease I would try this before consenting to a total colectomy.

Anorectal disease

In all **anorectal disease cancer should be ruled out** by proper physical exam (including proctosigmoidoscopic exam), even though the clinical presentation may suggest a specific benign process.

Hemorrhoids typically bleed when they are internal (can be treated with rubber band ligation), or hurt when they are external (may need surgery if conservative treatment fails). Internal hemorrhoids can become painful and produce itching if they are prolapsed.

Anal fissure happens to young women. They have exquisite pain with defecation and blood streaks covering the stools. The fear of pain is so intense that they avoid bowel movements (and get constipated) and sometimes refuse proper physical examination of the area. Exam may need to be done under anesthesia (the fissure is usually posterior, in the midline). A tight sphincter is believed to cause and perpetuate the problem, thus therapy is directed at relaxing it: stool softeners, topical nitroglycerin, local injection of botulinum toxin, forceful dilatation, or lateral internal sphincterotomy. Calcium channel blockers such as diltiazem ointment 2% TID topically for 6 weeks have had an 80–90% success rate, as compared to only 50% success for botulinum toxin.

Crohn's disease often affects the anal area. It starts with a fissure, fistula, or small ulceration, but the diagnosis should be suspected when the area fails to heal and gets worse after surgical interventions (the anal area typically heals very well because it has excellent blood supply—failure to do so means Crohn's disease). Surgery, in fact, should not be done in Crohn's disease of the anus. A fistula, if present, could be drained with setons while medical therapy is underway. Remicade helps healing.

Ischiorectal abscess (perirectal abscess) is very common. Patient is febrile, with exquisite perirectal pain that does not let him sit down or have bowel movements. Physical exam shows all the classic findings of an abscess (rubor, dolor, calor, and tumor) lateral to the anus, between the rectum and the ischial tuberosity. Incision and drainage are needed, and cancer should be ruled out by proper examination during the procedure. If patient is severely diabetic, horrible necrotizing soft tissue infection may follow: Watch him closely.

Fistula-in-ano develops in some patients who have had an ischiorectal abscess drained. Epithelial migration from the anal crypts (where the abscess originated) and from the perineal skin (where the drainage was done) form a permanent tract. Patient reports fecal soiling and occasional perineal discomfort. Physical exam shows opening (or openings) lateral to the anus, a cordlike tract may be felt, and discharge may be expressed. Rule out necrotic and draining tumor, and treat with fistulotomy.

Squamous cell carcinoma of the anus is more common in HIV+, and in homosexuals with receptive sexual practices. Fungating mass grows out of the anus, metastatic inguinal nodes are often felt. Diagnose with biopsy. Treatment starts with Nigro chemoradiation protocol, followed by surgery if there is **residual tumor**. Currently the 5-week chemo-radiation protocol has a 90% success rate, so surgery rarely is required.

Gastrointestinal Bleeding

General statistics of GI bleeding show that 3 of 4 cases originate in the upper GI tract (from the tip of the nose to the ligament of Treitz). One of 4 originates in the colon or rectum, and very few arise from the jejunum and ileum. GI bleeding arising from the colon comes from angiodysplasia, polyps, diverticulosis, or cancer, all of which are diseases of old people. Even hemorrhoids become more common with age. Thus, when a young patient has GI bleeding, the odds are overwhelming that it comes from the upper GI tract. When an old patient bleeds, it could be from anywhere (an "equal opportunity bleeder"), as the upper GI is the most common source overall ($^3/_4$), but age makes that old patient a good candidate for lower GI bleeding. Statistics are helpful when the bleeding is per rectum, but they are not needed when patients vomit blood.

Vomiting blood always denotes a source within the upper GI (tip of the nose to the ligament of Treitz). The same is true when blood is recovered by NG tube in a patient who shows up with bleeding per rectum. The best next diagnostic test in that setting is upper GI endoscopy. Be sure to look at the mouth and nose first.

Melena (black, tarry stools) always indicates digested blood, thus it must originate high enough to undergo digestion. Start workup with upper GI endoscopy.

Red blood per rectum could come from anywhere in the GI tract (including upper GI, as it may have transited too fast to be digested). The first diagnostic maneuver if the patient is actively bleeding at the time is to pass an NG tube and aspirate gastric contents. If blood is retrieved, an upper source has been established (follow with upper endoscopy). If no blood is retrieved and the fluid is white (no bile), the territory from the tip of the nose to the pylorus has been excluded, but the duodenum is still a potential source. Upper GI endoscopy should follow. If no blood is recovered and the fluid is green (bile tinged), the entire upper GI (tip of the nose to ligament of Treitz) has been excluded, and there is no need for an upper GI endoscopy.

Active bleeding per rectum, when upper GI has been excluded, is more difficult to work up. Bleeding hemorrhoids should always be excluded first (anoscopy), but colonoscopy is not helpful during active bleeding (the oncoming blood obscures the field). There are two ways to go after the hemorrhoids have been excluded. Some practitioners proceed according to the estimated rate of bleeding. If it exceeds 2 mL/min (1 unit of blood every 4 hours), they do an angiogram, which has a very good chance of finding the source and may allow for angiographic embolization. If the bleeding is less than 0.5 mL/min, they wait until the bleeding stops and then do a colonoscopy. For the cases in-between, they may do a tagged red-cell study. If the tagged blood puddles somewhere, an angiogram may be productive. The curse of the tagged red-cell study is that it is a slow test. By the time it's finished, the patient is often no longer bleeding, and the subsequent angiogram is useless. In that case, at least there is some idea if the puddling is on the right or the left and could thus guide a potential "blind" hemicolectomy in the future. If the tagged red cells do not show up on the scan, a subsequent colonoscopy is planned. Some practitioners always begin with the tagged red-cell study, regardless of the estimated rate of bleeding.

Patients with a recent history of blood per rectum, but not actively bleeding at the time of presentation, should start workup with upper GI endoscopy if they are young (overwhelming odds); but if they are old they need both an upper and a lower GI endoscopy (at the same session).

Blood per rectum in a child should be from Meckel diverticulum. Start workup with technetium scan, looking for the ectopic gastric mucosa.

Massive upper GI bleeding in the stressed, multiple trauma, or complicated post-op patient is probably from stress ulcers. Endoscopy will confirm. Angiographic embolization is the best therapeutic option. Better yet, they should be avoided by maintaining the gastric pH above 4.

The Acute Abdomen

Acute abdominal pain can be caused by perforation, obstruction, and inflammatory or ischemic processes. Each of these groups has some common identifying characteristics.

Acute abdominal pain caused by perforation has sudden onset and is constant, generalized, and very severe. The patient is reluctant to move, and very protective of his abdomen. Except in the very old or very sick, impressive generalized signs of peritoneal irritation are found (tenderness, muscle guarding, rebound, silent abdomen). If present, free air under the diaphragm in upright x-rays confirms the diagnosis.

Perforated peptic ulcer is the most common example. Emergency surgery is needed.

Acute abdominal pain caused by obstruction of a narrow duct (ureter, cystic, or common) has sudden onset of very severe colicky pain, with typical location and radiation according to source. The patient moves constantly, seeking a position of comfort. There are few physical findings, and they are limited to the area where the process is.

Acute abdominal pain caused by inflammatory process has gradual onset and slow buildup (at the very least a couple of hours, more commonly 6 or 10 or 12 hours), it is constant, starts as ill-defined, eventually locates to the area where the problem is, and often has typical radiation patterns. There are physical findings of peritoneal irritation in the affected area, and (except for pancreatitis) systemic signs such as fever and leukocytosis.

Ischemic processes affecting the bowel are the only ones that combine severe abdominal pain with blood in the lumen of the gut.

Primary peritonitis should be suspected in the child with nephrosis and ascites, or the adult with ascites who has a "mild" generalized acute abdomen with equivocal physical findings, and perhaps some fever and leukocytosis. Cultures of the ascitic fluid will yield a single organism (in garden-variety acute abdomens, a multiplicity of organisms grow). Treat with antibiotics, not with surgery.

The treatment for a generalized acute abdomen is exploratory laparotomy, with no need to have a specific diagnosis as to the exact nature of the process. If it does not look like primary peritonitis (one of the exceptions), we only need to rule out things that may mimic an acute abdomen—myocardial ischemia (EKG, troponins), lower lobe pneumonia (chest x-ray), PE (immobilized patient)—or things that specifically do not require surgery—pancreatitis (amylase or lipase) and urinary stones (CT scan of abdomen).

Acute pancreatitis should be suspected in the alcoholic who develops an "upper" acute abdomen. The classic picture has rapid onset for an inflammatory process (a couple of hours), and the pain is constant, epigastric, radiating straight through to the back, with nausea, vomiting, and retching. Physical findings are relatively modest, found in the upper abdomen. Diagnose with serum or urinary amylase or lipase (serum from 12 to 48 hours, urinary from third to sixth day). CT if diagnosis is not clear. Treat with NPO, NG suction, IV fluids. (More details in pancreatic disease section.)

Biliary tract disease should be suspected in the fat woman in her 40s who has "fifty-five children," and who develops right upper quadrant abdominal pain. (More details will be given in the section on biliary tract.)

Ureteral stones produce sudden onset of colicky flank pain radiating to inner thigh and scrotum (or labia), sometimes with other urinary symptoms like urgency and frequency; and with microhematuria in the urinalysis. CT scan is the best diagnostic test. (More details will be given in the urology section.)

Acute diverticulitis is one of the very few inflammatory processes giving acute abdominal pain in the left lower quadrant (in women the tube and ovary are other potential sources). Patient is middle-age or beyond, there is fever, leukocytosis, physical findings of peritoneal irritation in the left lower quadrant, sometimes palpable tender mass. CT is diagnostic. Start treatment with NPO, IV fluids, and antibiotics. Most will cool down. About 90% of those who do not, have an abscess that can be drained percutaneously by the radiologist. The few that cannot will need emergency surgery. Any patient who has survived 2 episodes of acute diverticulitis should have elective surgical removal of the affected area before they get into trouble again.

Volvulus of the sigmoid is seen in old people. There are signs of intestinal obstruction and severe abdominal distention. X-rays are diagnostic, as they show air-fluid levels in the small bowel, very distended colon, and a huge air-filled loop in the right upper quadrant that tapers down toward the left lower quadrant with the shape of a "parrot's beak." Proctosigmoidoscopic exam with the old rigid instrument resolves the acute problem. Rectal tube is left in. Recurrent cases need elective sigmoid resection.

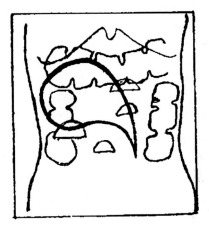

Volvulus of the sigmoid

Mesenteric ischemia is also seen predominantly in the elderly, but the real key is the development of an acute abdomen in someone with atrial fibrillation or a recent MI (the source of the clot that breaks off and lodges in the superior mesenteric artery). Because the very old do not mount impressive acute abdomens, often the diagnosis is made late, when there is blood in the bowel lumen (the only condition that mixes acute pain with GI bleeding) and acidosis and sepsis have developed. In very early cases, arteriogram and embolectomy might save the day.

Hepatobiliary

The liver

Primary hepatoma (hepatocellular carcinoma) is seen in the United States only in people with cirrhosis, or those known to have had hepatitis B or C. They develop vague right upper-quadrant discomfort and weight loss. The specific blood marker is α-fetoprotein. CT scan will show location and extent. Resection is done if technically possible.

Metastatic cancer of the liver outnumbers primary cancer of the liver in the United States by 20:1. They are found by CT scan if follow-up for the treated primary tumor is under way, or suspected because of rising carcinoembryonic antigen (CEA) in those who had colonic cancer. If the primary is slow growing and the metastases are confined to one lobe, resection can be done. Other means of control include radioablation.

Hepatic adenomas may arise as a complication of birth control pills and are important because they have a tendency to rupture and bleed massively inside the abdomen. CT scan is diagnostic, emergency surgery is required.

Pyogenic liver abscess is seen most often as a complication of biliary tract disease, particularly acute ascending cholangitis. Patients develop fever, leukocytosis, and a tender liver. Sonogram or CT scan are diagnostic. Percutaneous drainage is required.

Amebic abscess of the liver favors men, all of whom have a "Mexico connection." (It is very common there and seen here in immigrants.) Presentation and imaging diagnosis are similar, but this one can be treated with metronidazole, seldom requiring drainage. Definitive diagnosis is given by serology (the ameba does not grow in the pus), but because the test takes weeks to be reported, empiric treatment is started in those clinically suspected. If they improve, it is continued—if not, drainage is done.

Jaundice

Jaundice may be hemolytic, hepatocellular, or obstructive.

Hemolytic jaundice is usually low level (bilirubin of 6 or 8 . . . but not 35 or 40), and all the elevated bilirubin is unconjugated (indirect), with no elevation of the direct, conjugated fraction. There is no bile in the urine. Workup should determine what is chewing up the red cells.

Hepatocellular jaundice has elevation of both fractions of bilirubin and very high levels of transaminases, with modest elevation of the alkaline phosphatase. Hepatitis is the most common example, and workup should proceed in that direction (serologies to determine specific type).

Obstructive jaundice has elevations of both fractions of bilirubin, modest elevation of transaminases, and very high levels of alkaline phosphatase. First step in the workup is a sonogram, looking for dilatation of the biliary ducts, as well as further clues as to the nature of the obstructive process. In obstruction caused by stones, the stone that is obstructing the common duct is seldom seen, but stones are seen in the gallbladder, which because of chronic irritation cannot dilate. In malignant obstruction, a large, thin-walled, distended gallbladder is often identified (Courvoisier-Terrier sign).

Obstructive jaundice caused by stones should be suspected in the obese, fecund woman in her 40s who has high alkaline phosphatase, dilated ducts on sonogram, and nondilated gallbladder full of stones. The next move in that case is an endoscopic retrograde cholangiopancreatography (ERCP) to confirm the diagnosis, do sphincterotomy, and remove the common duct stone. Cholecystectomy should follow.

Obstructive jaundice caused by tumor is suggested by the thin-walled, dilated gallbladder in the sonogram. Three different cancers may be responsible: adenocarcinoma of the head of the pancreas, adenocarcinoma of the ampulla of Vater, or cholangiocarcinoma of the common duct itself. Significant weight loss and constant back pain suggest a large pancreatic tumor, which should be visible in a CT scan—the next test to run. In the absence of those clues or if the CT scan is negative, the next step is MRCP, which can show smaller tumors that are blocking the flow of bile thanks to strategic location— a cholangiocarcinoma, an ampullary cancer, or a small pancreatic malignancy abutting the intrapancreatic portion of the common duct. There are several options for the biopsy: CT-guided percutaneous for a large pancreatic mass, endoscopic for ampullary, ERCP and brushings for a ductal neoplasm, or endoscopic ultrasound for tiny tumors within the head of the pancreas.

ERCP or MRCP?

An endoscopic retrograde cholangiopancreatogram (ERCP) is an invasive procedure that allows visualization and instrumentation of the biliary and pancreatic ducts. An endoscope descends into the duodenum, the ampulla is cannulated, and x-ray dye is injected. Although experts can do all that in less than an hour, the need for sedation makes ERCP an all-day affair: nothing by mouth for several hours prior to the test; then the procedure itself; perhaps a bit of discomfort (gagging) if the sedation is light; and then a recovery period, after which the patient needs a ride home.

A newer study, magnetic resonance cholangiopancreatogram (MRCP) is completely noninvasive and is done on a fully awake patient. Every now and then it's necessary to hold breathing for about 10 seconds at a time, and the whole thing is over in roughly 10 minutes. No gagging, no limitations. Simple. And the pictures thus produced are gorgeous: detailed views of both ducts and the surrounding parenchyma.

Which of these two procedures should you subject your patients to?

Obviously, if all you need is a diagnostic picture, the clear choice is MRCP. But if you want to do more than look at a picture, you will need the ERCP. With the latter you can do sphincterotomies, retrieve stones, drain pus, deploy stents, biopsy tumors, and so on. Introduced as a diagnostic study only, ERCP has evolved into an instrument for therapy—which MRCP cannot do.

And sometimes a progressive sequence will make sense: Get your diagnosis and make your plans with the 10-minute, noninvasive test (MRCP). Then, if the findings call for manipulations, schedule the all-day affair (ERCP).

Ampullary cancers may be suspected when malignant obstructive jaundice coincides with anemia and positive blood in the stools. Ampullary cancer can bleed into the lumen like any other mucosal malignancy, at the same time that it can obstruct biliary flow by virtue of its location. Given that combination, endoscopy should be the first test.

Pancreatic cancer is seldom cured, even when the huge Whipple operation (pancreatoduodenectomy) is done. Ampullary cancer and cancer of the lower end of the common duct have a much better prognosis (about 40% cure). Cholangiocarcinomas that arise within the liver at the bifurcation of the hepatic ducts have terrible prognosis by virtue of their extremely inconvenient location. They can be beautifully shown by magnetic resonance cholangiopancreatography (MRCP), but achieving margin-free resection is almost impossible.

The gallbladder

Gallstones are responsible for the vast majority of biliary tract pathology. There is a spectrum of biliary disease caused by gallstones, as noted below. Although the obese woman in her 40s is the "textbook" victim, incidence increases with age so that eventually they are common in everybody, particularly Mexican Americans and Native Americans.

Asymptomatic gallstones are left alone.

Biliary colic occurs when a stone temporarily occludes the cystic duct. There is colicky pain in the right upper quadrant, radiating to the right shoulder and beltlike to the back, often triggered by ingestion of fatty food, accompanied by nausea and vomiting but without signs of peritoneal irritation or systemic signs of inflammatory process. The episode is self-limited (10, 20, maybe 30 minutes) or easily aborted by anticholinergics. If sonogram establishes diagnosis of gallstones, elective cholecystectomy is indicated.

Acute cholecystitis starts as a biliary colic, but the stone remains at the cystic duct until an inflammatory process develops in the obstructed gallbladder. Pain becomes constant, there is modest fever and leukocytosis, and there are physical findings of peritoneal irritation in the right upper quadrant. Liver function tests are minimally affected. Sonogram is diagnostic in most cases (gallstones, thick-walled gallbladder, and pericholecystic fluid). Rarely, a radionuclide scan (HIDA) might be needed (would show uptake in the liver, common duct, and duodenum, but not in the occluded gallbladder). NG suction, NPO, IV fluids, and antibiotics "cool down" most cases, allowing elective cholecystectomy to follow. Physicians typically endeavor to do it in the same hospital admission, as an urgent case, though it is not a "middle of the night" true emergency. If the patient does not respond (men and diabetics often do not), emergency cholecystectomy is needed. Emergency percutaneous transhepatic cholecystostomy may be the best temporizing option in the very sick with prohibitive surgical risk.

Acute ascending cholangitis is a far more deadly disease, in which stones have reached the common duct producing partial obstruction and ascending infection. Patients are often older and much sicker. Temperature spikes to 104°–105°F, with chills, and very high white blood cell (WBC) count indicate sepsis. There is some hyperbilirubinemia, but the key finding is extremely high levels of alkaline phosphatase. IV antibiotics and emergency decompression of the common duct (ideally by ERCP, alternatively percutaneous through the liver by percutaneous transhepatic cholangiogram [PTC], or rarely by surgery) are lifesaving. Eventually cholecystectomy has to follow.

Obstructive jaundice without ascending cholangitis can occur when stones produce complete biliary obstruction, rather than partial obstruction. Presentation and management were detailed in the jaundice section.

Surgical injuries to the biliary tract are devastating complications, with lifelong adverse consequences, due to the tendency of those structures to stricture as they heal.

Biliary pancreatitis is seen when stones become impacted distally in the ampulla, temporarily obstructing both pancreatic and biliary ducts. The stones often pass spontaneously, producing a mild and transitory episode of cholangitis along with the classic manifestations of pancreatitis (elevated amylase or lipase). Sonogram confirms gallstones in the gallbladder. Conservative treatment (NPO, NG suction, IV fluids) usually leads to improvement, allowing elective cholecystectomy to be done later. If not, ERCP and sphincterotomy may be required to dislodge the impacted stone.

The Pancreas

Acute pancreatitis is seen as a complication of gallstones (as described above) or in alcoholics. Acute pancreatitis may be edematous, hemorrhagic, or suppurative (pancreatic abscess). Late complications include pancreatic pseudocyst and chronic pancreatitis.

Acute edematous pancreatitis occurs in the alcoholic or the patient with gallstones. Epigastric and midabdominal pain starts after a heavy meal or bout of alcoholic intake, is constant, radiates straight through to the back, and is accompanied by nausea, vomiting, and (after the stomach is empty) continued retching. There is tenderness and mild rebound in the upper abdomen. Elevated serum amylase or lipase (early on) or urinary amylase or lipase (after a couple of days) are diagnostic, and a key finding to establish the edematous nature is an elevated hematocrit. Resolution usually follows a few days of pancreatic rest (NPO, NG suction, IV fluids).

Acute hemorrhagic pancreatitis is a much more deadly disease. It starts as the edematous form does, but an early laboratory clue is lower hematocrit (the degree of amylase elevation does not correlate with the severity of the disease). Other findings have been catalogued (Ranson's criteria), and they include at the time of presentation elevated WBC count, elevated blood glucose, and low serum calcium. By the next morning, the hematocrit is even lower, the serum calcium remains low (in spite of calcium administration), the blood urea nitrogen (BUN) goes up, and metabolic acidosis and low arterial PO_2 eventually are evident. Prognosis at that time is bad, and very intensive supportive therapy is needed (in the ICU). A common final pathway for death is the development of multiple pancreatic abscesses, and to anticipate them and drain them, if at all possible, daily CT scans are recommended. Carbapenems, quinolones, and metronidazole are known to penetrate infected necrotic pancreas, and they may be used prior to surgical drainage.

Pancreatic abscesses come to surgical attention via imaging studies, or when fever and leukocytosis develop about 10 days after the onset of pancreatitis. Ideally percutaneous radiological drainage should be performed. Because that is not always possible, open drainage may be required.

Necrosectomy may be the best way to deal with necrotic pancreas. This operation is best done when the dead tissue is well delineated, typically after 4 weeks. The material is "scooped out." The procedure may have to be repeated until all the dead matter has been cleared away.

Pancreatic pseudocyst can be a late sequela of acute pancreatitis or of pancreatic (upper abdominal) trauma. In either case about 5 weeks elapses between the original problem and the discovery of the pseudocyst. There is a collection of pancreatic juice outside the pancreatic ducts (most commonly in the lesser sac) and the pressure symptoms thereof (early satiety, vague discomfort, a deep palpable mass). Either CT or sonogram will be diagnostic. Treatment is dictated by the size and age of the pseudocyst. Cysts 6 cm or smaller, or those that have been present for less than 6 weeks are not likely to have complications and can be observed for spontaneous resolution. Bigger (>6 cm) or older cysts (>6 wk) are more likely to rupture or bleed, and they need to be treated. Treatment involves drainage of the cyst. The cyst can be drained percutaneously to the outside, drained surgically into the gastrointestinal tract, or drained endoscopically into the stomach.

Chronic pancreatitis is a devastating disease. People who have repeated episodes of pancreatitis (usually alcoholic) eventually develop calcified burned-out pancreas, steatorrhea, diabetes, and constant epigastric pain. The diabetes and steatorrhea can be controlled with insulin and pancreatic enzymes, but the pain is resistant to most modalities of therapy and it wrecks sufferers' lives. If MRCP shows specific points of obstruction and dilatation, operations that drain the pancreatic duct may help.

A Primer of Surgical Oncology

There are 3 big families of malignant tumors, which arise from the 3 layers of the embryo: epithelial tumors, which come from the ectoderm; sarcomas, which originate in mesodermal tissue; and adenocarcinomas, which grow from the endoderm.

The *sine qua non* of a malignant tumor—what makes a cancer a cancer—is its ability to metastasize. After an initial period when the tumor is still localized, cancer cells eventually travel to other parts of the body and set up shop there. There are two ways they can do that: lymphatic spread to regional and more distant lymph nodes, and hematogenous migration to far-away organs. The latter are typically "the two L's and the two B's": liver, lung, brain, and bone.

Epithelial tumors and adenocarcinomas use both modes of spreading, with particular tumors showing preferences. Breast favors the two B's. Abdominal adenos often choose the liver. Sarcomas, on the other hand, typically ignore the lymph nodes and go only blood-borne—and they love the lungs.

Medical students often assume that cancer is a disease of old age. Sometimes it is. Cancers of the breast and lung, for instance, are seen very rarely in young people. But primary malignant tumors of bone occur almost exclusively in children, and some cancers have no particular preference. Thyroid cancer, for instance, can happen at any age.

(continued)

A Primer of Surgical Oncology (*Cont'd*)

Virtually all cancer deaths happen because of metastatic spread—thus the importance of early diagnosis and treatment while the tumor is still localized, the golden opportunity to cure it. We can treat localized cancer with surgery, radiation, or both. Once there are malignant cells throughout the body, we need systemic therapy, and it is less likely to succeed. There are 3 options available. By far the most commonly used is chemotherapy—that is, drugs that target rapidly dividing cells. Unfortunately, various normal tissues also turn over rapidly, and they get clobbered too: the lining of the GI tract, hair follicles, and bone marrow. Specific agents have other unpleasant side effects as well. Adriamycin damages the myocardium, bleomycin produces pulmonary fibrosis, cyclophosphamide irritates the bladder, and platinum-based agents are neurotoxic.

Hormonal manipulations can be used for testicular or breast cancer. In the latter, estrogen and progesterone receptors are routinely tested and the appropriate blocking agents used (tamoxifen or anastrozole).

The most recent addition to the oncological armamentarium is immunotherapy. While the 2 best-known agents are pembrolizumab and nivolumab, new drugs are approved by the FDA all the time. Immunotherapy is very specifically targeted. Genetic markers are the main criteria, but a wide range of other factors may be considered, including response to previous treatments. The list of side effects is often very long—not surprising, because once we unleash the immune system, it can turn against the human body itself. While dramatic cures are widely publicized, more often than not all we get is a modest prolongation of life: a few months at best.

Diseases of the Breast

In all breast disease, cancer must be ruled out even if the presentation suggests benign disease. The only sure way to rule out cancer is to get tissue for the pathologist. Age correlates best with the odds for cancer: virtually unknown in the teens, rare in young women, quite possible by middle age, and very likely in the elderly. The much-quoted statement "One of every 8 women in the United States will develop breast cancer" is true only for those who have reached the age of 85. Women with family history are at risk from an earlier age. When breast cancer arises in young women, it tends to be very aggressive.

Mammography is not a substitute for tissue diagnosis but an adjunct to physical examination. Breast masses that may be missed by palpation may be seen in x-rays, and vice versa. As a regular screening exam, mammography should be started at age 40 (earlier if there is family history). Mammograms are not done before age 20 (breast is too dense) or during lactation (all you see is milk), but they can be done if needed during pregnancy. Mammographically or sonographically guided multiple core biopsies have become the most convenient, effective, and inexpensive way to biopsy breast masses, whether they are palpable or are discovered by screening mammogram.

Women who inherit the BRCA gene need early and frequent screening, but it should be done with MRIs rather than mammograms, which are carcinogenic if repeated frequently. Furthermore, past the age of 30 they should consider prophylactic bilateral mastectomies if they have the BRCA2 mutation, and that plus oophorectomies if they have the BRCA1 mutation.

Fibroadenomas are seen in young women (late teens, early 20s) as a firm, rubbery mass that moves easily with palpation. Either fine-needle aspiration (FNA) or sonogram is sufficient to establish diagnosis. Removal is optional (most women want them out, and we are happy to oblige).

Cystosarcoma phyllodes is seen in the late 20s. They grow over many years, becoming very large, replacing and distorting the entire breast, yet not invading or becoming fixed. Most are benign, but they have potential to become outright malignant sarcomas. Core or incisional biopsy is needed (FNA is not sufficient), and removal is mandatory.

Mammary dysplasia (fibrocystic disease, cystic mastitis) is seen in the 30s and 40s (goes away with menopause), with bilateral tenderness related to menstrual cycle (worse in the last 2 weeks) and multiple lumps that seem to come and go (they are cysts) also following the menstrual cycle. If there is no "dominant" or persistent mass, mammogram is all that is needed, but if there is a persistent mass (presumably a cyst but potentially a tumor), further steps are required. Aspiration is done (not FNA, but aspiration with a bigger needle and syringe). If clear fluid is obtained and the mass goes away, that's it. If the mass persists or recurs after aspiration, formal biopsy is required. If bloody fluid is aspirated, it should be sent for cytology.

Intraductal papilloma is seen in young women (20s to 40s) with bloody nipple discharge. Mammogram is needed to identify other potential lesions, but it will not show the papilloma (they are tiny). Galactogram may be diagnostic and guides surgical resection.

Breast abscess is seen only in lactating women (what appears to be a breast abscess at other times is cancer until proven otherwise). Incision and drainage is needed, but biopsy of the abscess wall should be part of the procedure.

Breast cancer should be suspected in any woman with a palpable breast mass, and the index of suspicion goes up with the patient's age. Other strong indicators of cancer include: ill-defined fixed mass, retraction of overlying skin, "orange peel" skin, recent retraction of the nipple, eczematoid lesions of the areola, reddish orange peel skin over the mass (inflammatory cancer), and palpable axillary nodes. A history of trauma does not rule out cancer.

Breast cancer during pregnancy is diagnosed exactly as if pregnancy did not exist and is treated the same way except for: no radiotherapy or hormonal manipulations at any time during the pregnancy, and no chemotherapy during the first trimester. Termination of the pregnancy is not necessary.

The radiological appearance of breast cancer is an irregular, speculated mass with asymmetric density, architectural distortion, or fine microcalcifications that were not there in the previous mammogram.

Treatment of resectable breast cancer starts with either of 2 operations. Small lesions, located far away from the nipple and areola of a large breast, are removed within only a segment of the mammary gland. The operation is called lumpectomy, or segmental resection, and it must be followed by radiotherapy. Large tumors lying right under the nipple and areola, and occupying most of a small breast, require a simple total mastectomy and do not need subsequent radiation. If lymph nodes are not palpable in the axilla, either operation must include a sentinel node biopsy. If enlarged lymph nodes are palpable in the axilla, they are resected.

Infiltrating ductal carcinoma is the standard form of breast cancer. Inflammatory cancer is the only variant with much worse prognosis (and the need for pre-op chemotherapy). Other variants (lobular, medullary, mucinous) have slightly better prognosis and are treated the same way as the standard infiltrating ductal. Lobular has higher incidence of bilaterality, but not high enough to justify bilateral mastectomy.

Ductal carcinoma in situ cannot metastasize (thus no axillary sampling is needed) but has very high incidence of recurrence if only local excision is done. Total simple mastectomy is recommended for multicentric lesions throughout the breast; because of the possibility of missing an invasive focus in multicentric disease, many practitioners add a sentinel node biopsy in those. Lumpectomy followed by radiation is used if the lesion (or lesions) is confined to one quarter of the breast.

Inoperable cancer of the breast is treated with chemotherapy (may also add radiation), and sometimes it is rendered operable. Inoperability is based on local extent (not metastases).

Adjuvant systemic therapy should follow surgery in virtually all patients, particularly if axillary nodes are positive. Chemotherapy is used in most cases, and hormonal therapy is added if the tumor is receptor positive. Premenopausal women receive tamoxifen, and post-menopausal women receive anastrozole. Frail, old women with tumors that are not too aggressive may be offered hormonal therapy alone. Women who are positive for HER-2 receptors should be given trastu-zumab (Herceptin) along with chemotherapy; it should not be given alone. Trastuzumab is currently the most powerful drug we have for systemic breast cancer.

Persistent headache or back pain (with areas of localized tenderness) in women who recently had breast cancer suggests metastasis. MRIs are diagnostic. Brain metastases can be radiated or resected. The vertebral pedicles are the favorite location in the spine.

Breast Cancer: An Example of Evolving Knowledge

My chairman at the Surgery Department used to say, "Half of everything that is written in our medical textbooks, is wrong. The problem is, we do not know which half."

We used to think that breast cancer spread in a step-by-step fashion: moving first to the nearest lymph nodes, then to more distant ones, and finally going blood-borne. Thus, we designed and executed ever more radical operations to "cure" the cancer while it was still at the lymphatic spread stage. We now know that when lymph nodes have cancer cells, "the cat is out of the bag." The whole body has little clumps of tumor, too small to be seen but no longer amenable to surgical resection. Axillary nodes have become a marker: They tell

(continued)

Breast Cancer: An Example of Evolving Knowledge (*Cont'd*)

us that systemic therapy is needed. Nowadays if we choose to clean out an axilla that is full of cancer, we are only debulking. We are making the job of the chemo and hormonal therapy a little easier by reducing the number of cells they have to kill.

Mammography as a preventive program is another topic that is full of myths. Even the age when we start to do it (should it be 40 years old, or 50?) was established by powerful female members of Congress rather than by scientific evidence. When evidence has been rigorously applied, estimates say that every life truly saved by those x-rays costs about $1 million. Not exactly a bargain . . . and a reason why you don't see government-financed mammogram programs in Bangladesh or Outer Mongolia.

Breast cancer in pregnant women is yet another classic example of evolving knowledge. It behaves aggressively. Thus, we used to recommend termination of the pregnancy. Until we realized that it was not the pregnancy that made those cancers nasty, but rather, the age of the patients. (By a remarkable coincidence, none of those pregnant women with breast cancer was in her 70s or 80s.)

Even the names we give to breast disease can have unexpected adverse effects. Look at "ductal carcinoma in situ"—an oxymoron if there was ever one. What makes a cancer a cancer is its ability to metastasize. But the way we manage this disease is based on the fact that it does not have that capability. *So why do we call it a cancer?* Thanks to the name, those women are denied insurance, employment, and peace of mind. Downright stupid.

Well, I have just told you that half of the information in this pocket-book is wrong. Does that make my little set of notes useless? No. I do not know which half of my chapters and paragraphs will turn out to be inaccurate. But neither do the people who write the exam questions.

Diseases of the Endocrine System

Most **thyroid nodules** are benign, but the few that are malignant must be diagnosed and treated. These can occur at any age, and the most worrisome item in the history would be prior exposure of the gland to radiation. As a rule, thyroid cancer does not affect thyroid function. Some practitioners start the workup with sonogram, which can exclude some lumps that are clearly not neoplastic. Otherwise the diagnosis is made by fine needle aspiration (FNA), which in most cases indicates whether the node is benign (if so, follow up) or has papillary, medullary, or anaplastic cancer. Follicular cancer is not easily diagnosed by FNA, and a lobectomy may be needed to determine if a follicular neoplasm is benign (adenoma) or malignant. Papillary cancer is very slow growing, and the extent of surgical resection is dictated by the size of the tumor or the presence of metastatic nodes. Follicular cancer has rudimentary function: It can take radioactive iodine if it does not have to compete with normal thyroid tissue. Thus, a total thyroidectomy is always done for follicular cancer, because doing so permits use of radioactive iodine in the future to identify and treat any potential metastasis. Medullary cancer comes from the C cells that make calcitonin (useful for follow-up). It is aggressive, and radical surgery is justified. Workup for pheochromocytoma is indicated, as they often coexist (MEN, type 2). Anaplastic cancer is seen in old people. It grows like wildfire, and often all that can be done for the patient is a tracheostomy.

Hyperthyroidism is treated with radioactive iodine in most cases. There is a very limited role for surgery on patients who have a "hot adenoma."

Hyperparathyroidism is most commonly found by serendipitous discovery of high serum calcium in blood tests (rarely seen in the full florid "disease of stones, bones, and abdominal groans"). Repeat calcium determinations, look for low phosphorus, and rule out cancer with bone metastases. If findings persist, do parathyroid hormone (PTH) determination (and interpret in light of serum calcium levels).

Help from Nuclear Medicine

I love the nuclear medicine people. They greatly facilitate my surgical work, particularly in the areas of endocrine surgery and surgical hypertension. They have identified substances that various glands in the body capture and use in their metabolic activity. They make those substances radioactive, so that when injected into a patient they are visible in a subsequent scan that reveals not only where they are but also how hard the glands are working.

A prime example is parathyroid surgery. People are supposed to have 4 parathyroid glands, all in the neck. A few weird characters have only 3, or perhaps 5. And there are truly perverted patients who have them in the mediastinum. Surgery for those used to be a nightmare. Not anymore. Sestamibi scans will give you the road map.

Pheochromocytomas are another example. They arise from chromaffin tissue. If they make epinephrine, the more refined end-product, pheochromocytomas are typically in the adrenal medulla. But those making the more primitive norepinephrine can be located anywhere from the base of the skull to the pelvis, on either side of the spine. A nuclear scan can identify them.

Finding pathological tissue is not all. Destroying it is another task that can be done with radioactive material—for instance, follicular cancer of the thyroid. Once all normal thyroid has been surgically removed, tumor mets become the best iodine trappers. A small tracer dose will identify those, and a bigger therapeutic one will kill them.

Scans work best in elective situations. It takes time to get the isotopes and to schedule their use. People bleeding to death somewhere inside the GI tract are not the best candidates. I know that many physicians like to use tagged red cell studies for those, but I prefer to rely on my estimation of the rate of bleeding. It's a lot quicker. Or, as I tell my students in jest: There are clocks on the walls all over the hospital, but in the nuclear medicine area, they have calendars instead.

Asymptomatic patients become symptomatic at a rate of 20% per year; thus elective intervention is justified. Ninety percent have single adenoma. Removal is curative. Sestamibi scan helps locate the offending gland or glands, and intraoperative PTH assay confirms that they have been extirpated. In the few patients who have hyperplasia, transplantation of all the parathyroids to the forearm facilitates future titration to keep the disease under control.

Cushing can be identified at a glance by looking at the picture of a lovely young woman next to a picture of a "monster" who is the same lady a couple of years later. The "monster" has a round, ruddy, hairy face, buffalo hump, supraclavicular fat pads, obese trunk with abdominal stria, and thin weak extremities. Osteoporosis, diabetes, hypertension, and mental instability are also present. Workup starts with an overnight low-dose dexamethasone suppression test. Suppression at low dosage rules out the disease (she is just a fat hairy lady). If there is no suppression, 24-hour urine-free cortisol is measured, and if elevated, we go to a high-dose suppression test. Suppression at a higher dose identifies pituitary microadenoma. No suppression at either dosage identifies adrenal adenoma (or paraneoplastic syndrome). Do appropriate imaging studies (MRI for pituitary, CT scan for adrenal) and remove the offending adenoma.

The Mayo Clinic advocates a different diagnostic algorithm, where the diagnosis of Cushing disease is established by 24-hour urinary collection for free cortisol levels (patients with this disease have levels 3–4 times the normal) and relies on measurement of corticotropin to differentiate pituitary adenomas from adrenal adenomas.

Zollinger-Ellison (gastrinoma) shows up as virulent peptic ulcer disease, resistant to all usual therapy (including eradication of *Helicobacter pylori*) and more extensive than it should be (several ulcers rather than one, ulcers extending beyond first portion of the duodenum). Some patients also have watery diarrhea. Measure gastrin and do secretin test if values are equivocal, locate the tumor with

CT scan (with contrast) of the pancreas and nearby areas. Remove it. Omeprazole helps those with metastatic disease.

Insulinoma produces CNS symptoms because of low blood sugar, always when the patient is fasting. Differential diagnosis is with reactive hypoglycemia (attacks occur after eating) and with self-administration of insulin. In the latter the patients have reason to be familiar with insulin (some connection with the medical profession, or with a diabetic patient), and in plasma assays they have high insulin but low C-peptide. In insulinoma both are high. Do CT (with contrast) of pancreas to locate tumor, and remove it. Some medically sophisticated patients are using sulfonylureas to induce endogenous insulin secretion, and defeat the diagnostic value of C-peptide. Levels of those drugs need to be measured in the workup.

Nesidioblastosis is a devastating hypersecretion of insulin in the newborn, requiring 95% pancreatectomy.

Glucagonoma produces severe migratory necrolytic dermatitis, resistant to all forms of therapy, in a patient with mild diabetes, a touch of anemia, glossitis, and stomatitis. Glucagon assay is diagnostic, CT scan is used to locate the tumor, resection is curative. Somatostatin and streptozocin can help those with metastatic, inoperable disease.

Surgical Hypertension

Primary hyperaldosteronism can be caused by an adenoma or by hyperplasia. In both cases the key finding is hypokalemia in a hypertensive (usually female) patient who is not on diuretics. Other findings include modest hypernatremia and metabolic alkalosis. Aldosterone levels are high, whereas renin levels are low. Appropriate response to postural changes (more aldosterone when upright than when lying down) suggests hyperplasia (which is treated medically), whereas lack of response (or inappropriate response) is diagnostic of adenoma. Adrenal CT scans localize it, and surgical removal provides cure.

Pheochromocytoma is typically seen in thin, hyperactive women who have attacks of pounding headache, perspiration, palpitations, and pallor (at which time they have extremely high blood pressure). By the time patients are seen, the attack has subsided and the pressure may be normal, leading to a very frustrating lack of diagnosis. Patients who have sustained hypertension are easier to diagnose. Start workup with 24-hour urinary determination of vanillylmandelic acid (VMA—easy to do, but may give false positives), metanephrines (more specific), or free urinary catecholamines. Follow with CT scan of adrenal glands or radionuclide studies if looking for extraadrenal sites. Tumors are usually large. Surgery requires careful pharmacologic preparation with alpha-blockers.

Coarctation of the aorta may be recognized at any age, but patients typically are young and have hypertension in the arms, with normal pressure (or low pressure, or no clinical pulses) in the lower extremities. Chest x-ray shows scalloping of the ribs (erosion from large collateral intercostals). Spiral CT scan enhanced with intravenous dye (CT angio) is usually diagnostic. Surgical correction is curative.

Renovascular hypertension is seen in two very distinct groups: young women with fibromuscular dysplasia or old men with arteriosclerotic occlusive disease. In both groups hypertension is resistant to the usual medications, and a telltale faint bruit over the flank or upper abdomen suggests the diagnosis. Workup is multifactorial, but Duplex scanning of the renal vessels and CT angio have prominent roles. Therapy is imperative in the young women, usually balloon dilatation and stenting; but it is much more controversial in the old men who may have short life expectancy from the other manifestations of the arteriosclerosis.

Decoding the Operative Note:
The Names of Operations

The name of an operation typically begins with the name of the structure being operated on, and an ending that indicates what was done. Here is a list of those endings.

-tomy means to cut. You might think it means to look inside a part of the body, because you have heard about "laparotomies," "craniotomies," and so forth. But we have to do a *-tomy* to get in there, because human bodies do not come equipped with convenient zippers. If we cut a tendon, that is a "tenotomy." If we slice open a fistula so it can fill in and heal, that is a "fistulotomy." And so on.

-ectomy means to take out or to resect, as in "appendectomy" or "cholecystectomy." Where there are different extents of what comes out, the name specifies it clearly: We can do total gastrectomies, subtotals, or hemigastrectomies. Or a right hemicolectomy, as opposed to a left hemicolectomy. Enough said.

-ostomy means to make a mouth; to make an opening. But this one is tricky. If the name of a single organ precedes the suffix *-ostomy*, the opening is to the outside, as in colostomy or "ileostomy." It could be done directly or by means of a tube or a cannula, as in "gastrostomy tube" or "tracheostomy." But if the names of two organs precede the ending, the opening is *between them*. It is an anastomosis. In the GI tract, anastomosis is always designated in the normal anatomical sequence, as in "gastrojejunostomy." Medical students trip on this one all the time. They read, "A patient had a right hemicolectomy and an ileotransverse colostomy," but they retain only the last word and start looking for the colostomy bag. There isn't one. The ileum was anastomosed to the transverse colon.

(*continued*)

Decoding the Operative Note:
The Names of Operations (*Cont'd*)

-plasty means to change the shape of something. Virtually all the cosmetic plastic surgery procedures are *-plasties*, but we also do them for functional reasons. For instance, a "pyloroplasty" enlarges the outlet of the stomach; an "annuloplasty" brings the leaflets of the mitral valve closer to each other, so the valve can close.

-pexy means to fix in place. For instance, "orchiopexy" affixes an undescended testicle where it should be. Many times we pile up a ton a procedures as part of a single operation. For instance we might do a "hemigastrectomy" with a "gastroduodenostomy" and, to provide decompression, add a "tube gastrostomy"; but fearing complications if the tube is dislodged, we add a "gastropexy."

-rrhaphy means to suture or sew together. "Herniorrhaphy" is the classic example for historical reasons, because surgeons used to sew up layers and layers of groin tissues to fix hernias. Today we often just laparoscopically put in a patch of plastic material. So here is another example: When ophthalmologists do fancy stuff that they want to protect from exposure to the outside, they add a "tarsorrhaphy": They sew up the eyelids together.

-scopic implies that an operation, or part of it, was done in a minimally invasive fashion using a TV camera inserted into a body cavity and several probes that do the actual operative steps. The term is derived from *-scope*, which means "to see."

Chapter 5
Pediatric Surgery

Birth Through the First 24 Hours

Most congenital anomalies require surgical correction, but in many of them other anomalies have to be looked for first. In some cases clusters are seen.

Esophageal atresia shows up with excessive salivation noted shortly after birth, or choking spells when first feeding is attempted. A small NG tube is passed, and it will be seen coiled in the upper chest when x-rays are done. If there is normal gas pattern in the bowel, the baby has the most common form of the four types, in which there is a blind pouch in the upper esophagus and a fistula between the lower esophagus and the tracheobronchial tree. Before therapy is undertaken, associated anomalies (the vertebral, anal, cardiac, tracheal, esophageal, renal, and radial [VACTER] constellation) have to be ruled out: Look at the anus for imperforation, check the x-ray for vertebral and radial anomalies, do echocardiogram looking for cardiac anomalies, and sonogram looking for renal anomalies. Primary surgical repair is preferred, but if it has to be delayed, a gastrostomy has to be done to protect the lungs from acid reflux.

Imperforate anus may be the clinical presentation (noted on physical exam) for the VACTER collection of anomalies. If so, the others have to be ruled out as detailed above. For the imperforate anus itself, look for a fistula nearby (to vagina or perineum). If present, repair can be delayed until further growth (but before toilet training time). If not, a colostomy needs to be done for high rectal pouches (and later the repair), or a primary repair can be done right away if the blind pouch is almost at the anus. The level of the pouch is determined with x-rays taken upside down (so that the gas in the pouch goes up), with a metal marker taped to the anus.

Congenital diaphragmatic hernia is always on the left, and the bowel will be up in the chest. The real problem is not the mechanical one, but the hypoplastic lung that still has fetal-type circulation. Repair must be delayed 3 or 4 days to allow maturation. Babies are in respiratory distress and need endotracheal intubation, low-pressure ventilation (careful not to blow up the other lung), sedation, and NG suction. Prenatal sonogram is diagnostic. Very severe cases that do not respond to conventional therapy are treated with extracorporeal membrane oxygenation (ECMO). The patients in these cases are children who would otherwise die, a circumstance that justifies this very expensive procedure. But ECMO is not a panacea in this setting. Early mortality from neurological complications, including intracranial bleeding, is very high, and the long-term health of the survivors is uncertain. Some have experienced continued pulmonary function deterioration and severe developmental problems.

Gastroschisis and omphalocele show up with an abdominal wall defect in the middle of the belly. In gastroschisis the cord is normal (it reaches the baby), the defect is to the right of the cord, there is no protective membrane, and the bowel looks angry and matted. In omphalocele the cord goes to the defect, which has a thin membrane under which one can see normal-looking bowel and a little slice of liver. Small defects can be closed primarily, but large ones require construction of a Silastic "silo" to house and protect the bowel. The contents of the silo are then squeezed into the belly, a little bit every day, until complete closure can be done in about a week. Babies with gastroschisis also need vascular access for parenteral nutrition, because the angry-looking bowel will not work for about 1 month.

Exstrophy of the urinary bladder is also an abdominal wall defect, but over the pubis (which is not fused), with a medallion of red bladder mucosa, wet and shining with urine. The baby has to be transferred immediately to a specialized center where a repair can be done within the first 1 or 2 days of life. Delayed repairs do not work.

Green vomiting in the newborn has ominous significance.

Green vomiting and a "double-bubble" picture in x-rays (a large air-fluid level in the stomach, and a smaller one to its right in the first portion of the duodenum) are found in **duodenal atresia, annular pancreas, or malrotation**. All of these anomalies require surgical correction, but malrotation is the most dangerous because the bowel can twist on itself, cut off its blood supply, and die. If in addition to the double bubble there is a little normal gas pattern beyond, the chances of malrotation are higher. Malrotation is diagnosed with contrast enema (safe, but not always diagnostic) or upper GI study (more reliable, but more risky). Although described here as a problem of the newborn, the first signs of malrotation can show up at any time within the first few weeks of life.

Intestinal atresia also shows up with green vomiting, but instead of a double bubble there are multiple air-fluid levels throughout the abdomen. There may be more than one atretic area, but no other congenital anomalies have to be suspected because this condition results from a vascular accident in utero.

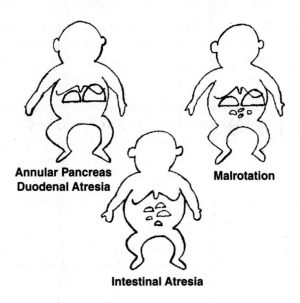

Annular Pancreas
Duodenal Atresia

Malrotation

Intestinal Atresia

A Few Days Old Through the First Two Months of Life

Necrotizing enterocolitis is seen in premature infants when they are first fed. There is feeding intolerance, abdominal distention, and a rapidly dropping platelet count (in babies, a sign of sepsis). Treatment: stop all feedings and administer broad-spectrum antibiotics, IV fluids, and IV nutrition. Surgical intervention is required if the infant develops abdominal wall erythema, air in the portal vein, intestinal pneumatosis (presence of gas in the bowel wall), or pneumoperitoneum (signs of intestinal necrosis and perforation).

Meconium ileus is seen in babies who have cystic fibrosis (often hinted at by the mother having it). They develop feeding intolerance and bilious vomiting. X-rays show multiple dilated loops of small bowel and a ground-glass appearance in the lower abdomen. Gastrografin enema is both diagnostic (microcolon and inspissated pellets of meconium in the terminal ileum) and therapeutic (Gastrografin draws fluid in, dissolves the pellets).

Hypertrophic pyloric stenosis shows up at age 3 weeks, more commonly in firstborn boys, with nonbilious projectile vomiting after each feeding. The baby is hungry and eager to eat again after he vomits. By the time they are seen they are dehydrated, with visible gastric peristaltic waves and a palpable "olive-size" mass in the right upper quadrant. If the mass cannot be felt, a sonogram is diagnostic. Therapy begins with rehydration and correction of the hypochloremic, hypokalemic metabolic alkalosis, followed by Ramstedt pyloromyotomy or balloon dilatation.

Biliary atresia should be suspected in 6- to 8-week-old babies who have persistent, progressively increasing jaundice (which includes a substantial conjugated fraction). Do serologies and sweat test to rule out other problems, and do HIDA scan after 1 week of phenobarbital (which is a powerful choleretic). If no bile reaches the duodenum even with phenobarbital stimulation, surgical exploration is needed. About one third can get a long-lasting surgical derivation, about one third need a liver transplant after they survived for a while with a surgical derivation, and about one third need the transplant right away.

Hirschsprung disease (aganglionic megacolon) can be recognized in early life or may go undiagnosed for many years. The cardinal symptom is chronic constipation. With short segments, rectal exam may lead to explosive expulsion of stool and flatus, with relief of abdominal distention. In older kids in whom differential diagnosis with psychogenic problems is an issue, presence of fecal soiling suggests the latter. X-rays show distended proximal colon (the normal one) and "normal-looking" distal colon, which is the aganglionic part. Diagnosis is made with full-thickness biopsy of rectal mucosa. Ingenious operations have been devised to preserve the unique sensory input of the motor-impaired rectum, while adding the normal propulsive capability of the innervated colon.

Later in Infancy

Intussusception is seen in 6- to 12-month-old chubby, healthy-looking kids who have episodes of colicky abdominal pain that makes them double up and squat. The pain lasts for about 1 minute, and the kid looks perfectly happy and normal until he gets another colic. Physical exam shows a vague mass on the right side of the abdomen, an "empty" right lower quadrant, and "currant jelly" stools. Barium or air enema is both diagnostic and therapeutic. If reduction is not achieved radiologically (or if there are recurrences), surgery is done.

Child abuse should always be suspected when injuries cannot be properly accounted for. Some classic presentations include subdural hematoma plus retinal hemorrhages (shaken baby syndrome), multiple fractures in different bones at different stages of healing, and all scalding burns, particularly burns of both buttocks (the child was held by arms and legs and dipped into boiling water).

Meckel diverticulum should be suspected in lower GI bleeding in the pediatric age group. Do radioisotope scan (technetium) looking for gastric mucosa in the lower abdomen.

Undescended testicle that has not reached the scrotum by the age of one needs to be surgically brought down there and fixed in place (orchiopexy). Note that a testicle that is in the canal at birth, but can be easily pulled down where it belongs, is not an undescended testicle; it is an overactive cremasteric muscle. Parents need to be reassured of the benign nature of the latter.

Abdominal masses in children are typically discovered by the mother. Mothers constantly handle their babies, are very familiar with their anatomy, and immediately recognize a change. If, on examination, the mass moves up and down with respiration, it is most likely a malignant liver tumor (hepatoblastoma or hepatocellular carcinoma). Alpha fetoprotein is likely to be elevated. If the mass is deeper and nonmobile, there is an even chance that it is a Wilms tumor arising from the kidney or a neuroblastoma growing in the adrenal gland.

Modern imaging devices (CT scan, MRI) can easily clarify what it is. Most of these malignancies are treated with surgical resection, if possible, and often they are subjected to additional chemotherapy or radiation. The prognosis in neuroblastoma depends on the child's age when it is discovered. The younger the patient is, the better the cure rate. A curious added feature of the neuroblastoma is that it may involute and spontaneously revert to a benign neuroma.

Childhood leukemia may be cured in the near future, if current trials with genetically modified immune cells (CAR T-cell therapy) are successful.

Fluid Needs in Children

When we assess basic, maintenance fluid needs in adults, we do not need formulas, calculators, or clever mnemonics. Adults need 2 to 3 liters per day. We simply eyeball the patients. A big fellow is a "3-liter-a-day person" and a tiny one is a "2-liter-a-day person."

But children are different. A newborn is much, much smaller than a teenager. Smaller creatures have more body surface area per unit of weight than bigger ones and, thus, greater fluid requirements. A formula is needed. Let me offer you one based on numbers that you carry in your pocket or purse: paper money.

There are U.S. bills in the following denominations: 1, 2, 5, 10, 20, 50, and 100. (I know two-dollar bills are rare, but they exist and are legal currency. They have a picture of Jefferson.) Take the middle of those seven numbers: 10. This handy formula specifies basic, maintenance fluid needs in increments of 10 kilograms: needs for the first 10 kg of body weight, then needs for the next 10 kg, and finally needs for everything above that weight (i.e., above 20 kg).

If you want to remember aliquots per day, look at the bigger bills: 100, 50, and 20. The pediatric patient should get 100 cc of fluid per kg of body weight per day up to 10 kg of body weight, plus 50 cc per kg

(continued)

Fluid Needs in Children (*Cont'd*)

of body weight per day for the next 10 kg of body weight, and finally another 20 cc per kg per day for anything above that weight (20 kg).

If you would rather think in terms of hourly administration, use the smaller denominations: 5, 2, and 1. Give babies 5 cc of liquids per kg per hour for the first 10 kg of body weight. A baby who weighs more than 10 kg gets another 2 cc per kg per hour. For a baby bigger than 20 kg, the rate goes down to 1 cc per kg per hour.

I know that the mathematics of what I have suggested are not precise. Days have 24 hours, not 20, and 2 is not half of 5. But these figures are good enough for our purposes.

Assessing basic, maintenance fluid needs per day helps you get the big picture. But one caution: Never order fluids "per day." Suppose you ask the nurses to give *x* amount in the next 24 hours and the IV immediately gets plugged up: Nothing happens for the first 23 hours, and then the full amount is pushed in a few minutes. Can you complain? No. You said you wanted *x* infused within 24 hours, and by God, that was done. None of that can happen if you always write your fluid orders specifying rate *per hour*.

I gave you this formula to use in children because you cannot simply eyeball pediatric patients and write basic, maintenance fluid orders that way. But the formula works for everybody. Recall that adults need 2 to 3 liters of liquids every day. Now apply the formula to figure out what the proverbial 70 kg person would get:

100 cc per kg per day for the first 10 kg of body weight: 1,000 cc.

Another 50 cc per kg per day for the next 10 kg: 500 cc.

And 20 cc per kg of body weight thereafter, in this case another 50 kg: 1,000 cc.

Total? 2,500 cc. Just what we knew all along.

CHAPTER 6
Cardiothoracic Surgery

Congenital Heart Problems

When a child has expiratory wheezing, it suggests bronchoconstriction, i.e., asthma. Inspiratory wheezing is seen in tracheomalacia, where the tracheal rings collapse. But if the parents report that the child has some difficulty swallowing, as well as episodes of respiratory distress, with crowing respiration, stridor, and hyperextension of the neck, the problem is **vascular ring**, a congenital anomaly in which the trachea and esophagus are encircled by abnormal blood vessels. Extrinsic compression is demonstrated by barium swallow and bronchoscopy. Surgery divides the smaller of the two aortic arches.

Morphologic cardiac anomalies (congenital or acquired) are best diagnosed with an echocardiogram.

Left-to-right shunts share the presence of a murmur, overloading of the pulmonary circulation, and long-term damage to the pulmonary vasculature. The volume and consequences of the shunt are different at different locations, as noted below.

Atrial septal defect has very minor, low-pressure, low-volume shunt. Patients typically grow into late infancy before it is recognized. A faint pulmonary flow systolic murmur and fixed split second heart sound are characteristic. A history of frequent colds is elicited. Echocardiogram is diagnostic. Closure can be achieved surgically or by cardiac catheterization.

Small, restrictive ventricular septal defects low in the muscular septum produce a heart murmur, but otherwise few symptoms. They are likely to close spontaneously within the first 2 or 3 years of life.

Ventricular septal defects in the more typical location (high in the membranous septum) lead to trouble early on. Within the first few months there will be "failure to thrive," a loud pansystolic murmur best heard at the left sternal border, and increased pulmonary vascular markings on chest x-ray. Do echocardiogram and surgical closure.

Patent ductus arteriosus becomes symptomatic in the first few days of life. There are bounding peripheral pulses and a continuous "machinery-like" heart murmur. Echocardiogram is diagnostic. In premature infants who have not gone into congestive heart failure, closure can be achieved with indomethacin. Those who do not close, those who are already in failure, or full-term babies need surgical division or radiological embolization with metal coils.

Right-to-left shunts share the presence of a murmur, diminished vascular markings in the lung, and cyanosis. Although 5 are always described (all beginning with the letter T), 3 of them are rather rare and will not be reviewed (one of them, truncus arteriosus, is fascinating because it is cyanotic but it kills by overloading the pulmonary circulation, like the noncyanotic shunts do). The common ones follow.

Tetralogy of Fallot, although crippling, often allows children to grow up into infancy. It is also the most common cyanotic anomaly, and thus any exam question in which a 5- or 6-year-old is cyanotic is bound to be tetralogy. The children are small for their age, have a bluish hue in the lips and tips of their fingers, clubbing, and spells of cyanosis relieved by squatting. There is a systolic ejection murmur in the left third intercostal space, a small heart, diminished pulmonary vascular markings on chest x-ray, and EKG signs of right ventricular hypertrophy. Echocardiogram is diagnostic, surgical repair is done.

Transposition of the great vessels leads to severe trouble early on. The kids are kept alive by an atrial septal defect, ventricular septal defect, or patent ductus (or a combination), but die very soon if not corrected. Suspect this diagnosis in a 1- or 2-day-old child with cyanosis who is in deep trouble, and ask for echocardiogram. The technical details of the surgical correction are mind-boggling, and you do not have to know them.

Acquired Heart Disease

Aortic stenosis produces angina and exertional syncopal episodes. There is a harsh midsystolic heart murmur best heard at the right second intercostal space and along the left sternal border. Start workup with echocardiogram. Surgical valvular replacement is indicated if there is a gradient of more than 50 mm Hg, or at the first indication of congestive heart failure, angina, or syncope.

Chronic aortic insufficiency produces wide pulse pressure and a blowing, high-pitched, diastolic heart murmur best heard at the second intercostal space and along the left lower sternal border, with the patient in full expiration. These patients are often followed with medical therapy for many years but should undergo valvular replacement at the first evidence on echocardiogram of beginning left ventricular dilatation.

Acute aortic insufficiency because of endocarditis is seen in young drug addicts who suddenly develop congestive heart failure and a new, loud diastolic murmur at the right second intercostal space. Emergency valve replacement and long-term antibiotics are needed.

Patients with a prosthetic valve need antibiotic prophylaxis for subacute bacterial endocarditis.

Mitral stenosis is caused by rheumatic fever many years before presentation. It produces dyspnea on exertion, orthopnea, paroxysmal nocturnal dyspnea, cough, and hemoptysis. There is a low-pitched, rumbling diastolic apical heart murmur. As it progresses, patients become thin and cachectic and develop atrial fibrillation. Workup starts with echocardiogram. As symptoms become more disabling, mitral valve repair becomes necessary with a surgical commissurotomy or a balloon valvuloplasty.

Mitral regurgitation is most commonly caused by valvular prolapse. Patients develop exertional dyspnea, orthopnea, and atrial fibrillation. There is an apical, high-pitched, holosystolic heart murmur that radiates to the axilla and back. Workup and surgical indications are as above, with repair of the valve (annuloplasty) preferred over prosthetic replacement.

Coronary disease can happen to anybody (including women), but the typical patient is a middle-aged sedentary man with a family history, a history of smoking, type 2 diabetes, and hypercholesterolemia. Progressive, unstable, disabling angina is the main reason to do cardiac catheterization and evaluate as a potential candidate for revascularization. Intervention is indicated if one or more vessels have 70% (or greater) stenosis and there is a good distal vessel. Preferably, the patient should still have good ventricular function (you cannot resuscitate dead myocardium). The general rule is the simpler the problem, the more it is amenable to angioplasty and stent; whereas more complex situations do better with surgery. Single vessel disease (that is not the left main or the anterior descending) is perfect for angioplasty and stent. Triple vessel disease makes multiple coronary bypass (using the internal mammary for the most important vessel) the best choice. Newer "hybrid" operating rooms that combine the facilities for heart surgery with the radiological equipment to do angioplasty increase flexibility to tailor the therapy for each specific patient. For example, the surgeons might hook up the internal mammary to the anterior descending, and then the interventional cardiologist might do angioplasty and stents on the other, less critical vessels.

Post-op care of heart surgery patients often requires that cardiac output be optimized. If cardiac output is considerably under normal (5 liters/min, or a cardiac index of 3), the pulmonary wedge pressure (or left atrial pressure, or left end-diastolic pressure) should be measured. Low numbers (zero to 3) suggest the need for more IV fluids. High numbers (20 or above) suggest ventricular failure.

The Lung

A coin lesion found on a chest x-ray has an 80% chance of being malignant in people over the age of 50, even higher if there is a history of smoking. A very expensive workup for cancer of the lung, however, can be avoided if an older (a year or two) chest x-ray shows the same unchanged lesion (it is not cancer). Thus, seeking an older x-ray is always the "first thing to do" in the patient found to have a coin lesion.

If no older chest x-ray is available, or the lesion was not present in a previous film, some practitioners want a biopsy to be done right away. However, it is prudent to do noninvasive studies before invasive ones, and thus I suggest that the next step should be sputum cytology and CT scan of the chest and upper abdomen (the latter to look for mets).

Diagnosis of cancer of the lung, if not established by cytology, requires bronchoscopy and biopsies (for central lesions) or percutaneous biopsy (for peripheral lesions). If those are unsuccessful, video-assisted thoracic surgery (VATS) and wedge resection may be needed. How far one goes in that sequence depends on the probability of cancer (higher in elderly with history of smoking and noncalcified lesion in CT), the assurance that surgery can be done (residual pulmonary function will suffice), and the chances that the surgery may be curative (no metastases to mediastinal or carinal nodes, the other lung, or the liver). The interplay of these three determines specific sequence of workup beyond sputum cytology and CT scan in each patient.

Small cell cancer of the lung is treated with chemotherapy and radiation, and therefore assessment of operability and curative chances of surgery are not applicable. Operability and possibility of surgical cure applies only to non–small cell cancer.

Operability of lung cancer is predicated on residual function after resection. (Assuming pneumonectomy is required. For lobectomy, function is less of an issue. Central lesions require pneumonectomy. Peripheral lesions can be removed with lobectomy.) A minimum FEV_1 of 800 mL is needed. If clinical findings (COPD, shortness of breath) suggest this may be the limiting factor, pulmonary function studies are done. Determine FEV_1, determine fraction that comes from each lung (by ventilation-perfusion scan), and figure out what would remain after pneumonectomy. If less than 800 mL, do not continue expensive tests. The patient is not a surgical candidate. Treat with chemotherapy and radiation.

Potential cure by surgical removal of lung cancer depends on extent of metastases. Hilar metastases can be removed with the pneumonectomy, but nodal metastases at the carina or mediastinum preclude curative resection. CT scan may identify nodal metastases, and more recently, the addition of PET scanning has helped define the presence of an actively growing tumor in enlarged nodes. Endobronchial ultrasound is a more invasive option to sample mediastinal nodes. Metastases to the other lung, the adrenal, or the liver should also be evident in the CT.

Treatment of non–small cell lung cancer has benefited from the recent introduction of immunotherapy. Both pembrolizumab and nivolumab are now options for selected patients.

CHAPTER 7
Vascular Surgery

Subclavian steal syndrome is rare but fascinating (medical school professors love it, thus it is likely to appear on exams). An arteriosclerotic stenotic plaque at the origin of the subclavian (before the takeoff of the vertebral) allows enough blood supply to reach the arm for normal activity, but does not allow enough to meet higher demands when the arm is exercised. When that happens, the arm sucks blood away from the brain by reversing the flow in the vertebral. Clinically the patient describes claudication of the arm (coldness, tingling, muscle pain) and posterior neurologic signs (visual symptoms, equilibrium problems) when the arm is exercised. Vascular symptoms alone would suggest thoracic outlet syndrome, but the combination with neurologic symptoms identifies the subclavian steal. Duplex scanning is diagnostic when it shows reversal of flow. Bypass surgery cures it.

Abdominal aortic aneurysm (AAA) is typically asymptomatic, found as a pulsatile abdominal mass on examination (between the xiphoid and the umbilicus) or found on x-rays, sonograms, or CT scans done for another diagnostic purpose, usually in an older man. Size is the key to management, and thus if the aneurysm was found by physical exam, sonogram or CT scan is needed to provide precise measurements. If the aneurysm is 4 cm or smaller, it can be safely observed and the chances of rupture are almost zero. If it is 5–6 cm or larger, the patient should have elective repair because the chance of rupture is very high. Aneurysms that grow 1 cm per year or faster also need elective repair. Those were traditionally done by open laparotomy, but about 70% of them are now performed by percutaneously inserted vascular stents.

Surgery for a ruptured abdominal aortic aneurysm carries very high morbidity and mortality, thus efforts are made to predict and anticipate rupture, and not wait for it to occur.

A tender abdominal aortic aneurysm is going to rupture within a day or two, and thus immediate repair is indicated.

Excruciating back pain in a patient with a large abdominal aortic aneurysm means that the aneurysm is already leaking. Retroperitoneal hematoma is already forming, and blowout into the peritoneal cavity is only minutes or hours away. Emergency surgery is required.

Arteriosclerotic occlusive disease of the lower extremities has an unpredictable natural history (except for the predictable negative impact of smoking), and therefore there is no role for "prophylactic" surgery. Surgery is done only to relieve disabling symptoms or to save the extremity from impending necrosis. The first clinical manifestation is pain brought about by walking and relieved by rest (intermittent claudication). If the claudication does not interfere significantly with the patient's lifestyle, no workup is indicated. Cessation of smoking, a program of exercise, and the use of cilostazol can help the patient in the long run.

The workup of disabling intermittent claudication starts with Doppler studies looking for a pressure gradient, also known as establishing an ankle-brachial index. If there isn't a gradient between blood pressure measured in the arm and at various places in the leg (an ankle-brachial index of 1), then the disease is in the small vessels and not amenable to surgery. If there is a significant gradient (ankle-brachial index of 0.8 or less), follow with CT angio or MRI angio to look at the anatomy and plan the revascularization. The MRI has the advantages of avoiding ionizing radiation and the nephrotoxicity of iodinated contrast material, which in some patients limit the use of the CT angio. An impressive array of interventions is now available. Bypasses, for which saphenous vein grafts are harvested from the patient and reversed, remain the most durable option. Obviously, large-diameter arteries require prosthetic materials. Angioplasty and stents, once reserved for short segments, have exploded as the most sophisticated current option for most patients. Stents can be impregnated with medication, hooked to each other, or composed of a nickel alloy with shape memory triggered by temperature. Presurgery, nickel alloy stents are stored in the freezer in the closed position. Once inserted percutaneously where they need to go, *voila!* The blood warms them, and they deploy by themselves. Like science fiction!

Rest pain is the penultimate stage of the disease (the ultimate is ulceration and gangrene). The clinical picture is rather characteristic. The patient seeks help because he "cannot sleep." It turns out that pain in the calf is what keeps him from falling asleep. He has learned that sitting up and dangling the leg helps the pain, and a few minutes after he does so, the leg that used to be very pale becomes deep purple. Physical exam shows shiny atrophic skin without hair, and no peripheral pulses. Workup and therapy are as detailed above.

Arterial embolization from a distant source is seen in patients with atrial fibrillation (a clot breaks off from the atrial appendage) or those with a recent MI (the source of the embolus is the mural thrombus). The patient suddenly develops a painful, pale, cold, pulseless, paresthetic, and paralytic lower extremity (if you substitute "poikilothermic" for "cold," you have all the "P"s that are the mnemonic). Urgent evaluation and treatment should be completed within 6 hours. Doppler studies will locate the point of obstruction. Early incomplete occlusion may be treated with clot busters. Embolectomy with Fogarty catheter is done for complete obstructions, and fasciotomy should be added if several hours have passed before revascularization.

Dissecting aneurysm of the thoracic aorta occurs in the poorly controlled hypertensive. The episode resembles an MI, with sudden onset of extremely severe, tearing chest pain that radiates to the back and migrates down shortly after its onset. There may be unequal pulses in the upper extremities, and x-ray shows a wide mediastinum. EKG and cardiac enzymes rule out MI. Definitive diagnosis should be sought by noninvasive means (to avoid high-pressure injection needed for the aortogram). MRI angiogram, if available as an emergency, provides the best diagnostic images. CT angiogram has often been used because of wide availability, but because of the nephrotoxicity of the contrast material, it should be avoided if the patient has limited renal function. A third option would be a transesophageal echocardiogram. As a rule (riddled with exceptions), dissections of the ascending aorta are treated surgically, whereas those in the descending are managed medically with control of the hypertension in the ICU. In the former, the aortic valve may have been damaged and thus may require repair. In the latter, the devastating consequences of interrupting the blood supply to the spinal cord make surgery a risky proposition, and it is rarely done.

The Riddle of Biopsies: FNA Versus Core, Incisional Versus Excisional

If we think that there is a cancer somewhere inside the body, we have two options to prove it. The easier one is fine needle aspiration (FNA). It can be done at the office, does not require local anesthetic, and poses virtually no risk. As the name implies, a very fine needle is inserted into the target, and cells are aspirated for a pathologist to look at. Sometimes we get lucky and are rewarded with a diagnosis in a very simple and inexpensive way. But this method denies the pathologist a view of the tissue architecture, so many times a diagnosis cannot be made. In that case, a "negative" answer does not signify no cancer. It is completely meaningless.

(continued)

The Riddle of Biopsies: FNA Versus Core, Incisional Versus Excisional (*Cont'd*)

I am aware of only two circumstances *when an FNA is contraindicated*:

1. Do not do an FNA if you think there is a hemangioma in the liver: Should the patient take a deep breath when the needle is in, it could slice the hemangioma, leading to fatal bleeding.

2. Do not do an FNA of a testicular mass. These are almost invariably malignant and will quickly spread through the needle tract.

Core biopsy uses a much thicker, hollow needle with an outer jacket and an inner piece. Local anesthetic is required. Preferably guided by imaging, the whole assembly is introduced to the target, then the inner piece is advanced further and the jacket is advanced over the inner piece. This traps a little cylinder of tissue that is retrieved for biopsy. The procedure may be repeated several times to enhance the diagnostic yield. Sometimes, however, vital structures are in the way, precluding the use of core biopsy.

When a suspected cancer is on the skin or otherwise accessible, our options are incisional versus excisional. The key criterion is the size of the lesion. Tiny ones can be removed in toto. On bigger ones we should only take a sample, by cutting a little piece, preferably at the edge of the lesion.

CHAPTER 8
Skin Surgery

Exposure to the sun is the main cause of skin cancers. The typical victim is a fair-skinned person who does not enjoy the protection afforded by melanin. The damage is cumulative. A patient who repeatedly had sunburns with blistering as a youngster is very likely to develop cancers in later years.

Basal cell carcinoma accounts for about 50% of these. Three features are typical: It favors the upper part of the face; it has a timetable measured in years; and it does not metastasize. It kills by relentless local invasion ("rodent ulcer"). It may look like a waxy, raised lesion, or it may be an ulcer. The former can be simply excised, for both diagnosis and treatment. The latter should be biopsied at the edge. Resection requires only a 1 mm margin all around. To assure cure and avoid unnecessary mutilation, a sophisticated method called Mohs surgery performs repeated microscopic sections as the excision is being done.

Squamous cell carcinoma represents 25% of skin cancers and prefers the lower lip and the rest of the body. It has a timetable measured in months, and it can metastasize to lymph nodes. The latter may need to be sampled and, if involved, removed. Surgical margins for the primary lesion should be 0.5–2 cm. Radiation therapy is another treatment option.

Melanoma is the most lethal of these tumors. Incidence is currently increasing from a long-quoted figure of 15% of skin cancers. It usually originates in a previously benign pigmented lesion. The mnemonic to recognize melanomas is ABCDE: They are asymmetrical (A), with irregular borders (B), different colors within the lesion (C), and a diameter exceeding 0.5 cm (D), or they have evolved (E), i.e., an existing pigmented lesion has undergone a sudden change in its usual appearance.

The prognosis and management of melanoma is determined by its depth of invasion. The details keep changing, but the basic idea is simple: Superficial lesions have good prognosis, deep ones do not. Melanomas less than 1 mm deep require only local excision. Deeper lesions require wide margins (2 cm) and attention to lymph nodes (biopsy and/or remove as needed), and those between 1 and 4 mm benefit the most from aggressive efforts. Lesions beyond 4 mm have a terrible prognosis regardless of therapy.

Metastatic malignant melanoma is a bizarre, unpredictable, and fascinating disease. It goes to the usual places (lymph nodes, liver, lung, brain, and bone), but it also is the all-time champion for metastasizing to weird places. Furthermore, it has no predictable timetable. Some patients are full of metastases and dead within a few months of diagnosis and treatment; others go 20 years or more between the original treatment and the sudden explosion of metastases.

Disseminated melanoma cannot be cured. Interferon offers a modest improvement in survival time, and thus has been the standard treatment. We now favor targeted therapy, which may be better: The tumor genes are studied and the best agent chosen. These include chemotherapy (dacarbazine) and immunotherapy (pembrolizumab). The latter is credited with dramatic improvement for former president Jimmy Carter, whose brain mets from melanoma melted away. No one claims that he was cured, though. In their own advertising, the manufacturers of pembrolizumab promise only "a chance to live longer."

CHAPTER 9
Ophthalmology

Children

Amblyopia is a vision impairment resulting from interference with the processing of images by the brain during the first 6 or 7 years of life. The most common expression of this phenomenon is the child with strabismus. Faced with two overlapping images, the brain suppresses one of them. If the strabismus is not corrected early on, there will be permanent cortical blindness of the suppressed eye, even though the eye is perfectly normal. Should an obstacle impede vision in one eye during those early years (for instance, a congenital cataract), the same problem will develop.

Strabismus is verified by showing that the reflection from a light comes from different areas of the cornea in each eye. Strabismus should be surgically corrected when diagnosed to prevent the development of amblyopia. When reliable parents relate that a child did not have strabismus in the early years but develops it later in infancy, the problem is an exaggerated convergence caused by refraction difficulties. In that case corrective glasses instantly resolve the problem. True strabismus does not resolve spontaneously.

A **white pupil in a baby** (leukocoria) is an ophthalmologic emergency, as it may be caused by a retinoblastoma. Even if the white pupil is caused by a less lethal problem, like a congenital cataract, it should be attended to in order to prevent amblyopia.

Adults

Glaucoma is a very common source of blindness, but because of its silent nature, it is unlikely to be discovered by regular physicians (or to be tested for in an exam). One variant, however, should be recognized by every physician who might encounter it. Acute angle closure glaucoma shows up as very severe eye pain or frontal headache, typically starting in the evening when the pupils have been dilated for several hours (watching a double feature at the movies, or watching TV in a dark room). The patient—often a female of Asian extraction—may report seeing halos around lights. On physical exam the pupil is mid-dilated and does not react to light, the cornea is cloudy with a greenish hue, and the eye feels "hard as a rock." Emergency treatment is required (ophthalmologists will drill a hole in the iris with a laser beam to provide a drainage route for the fluid that is trapped in the anterior chamber). While waiting for the ophthalmologist, administer systemic carbonic anhydrase inhibitors (such as Diamox) and apply topical beta-blockers and alpha-2–selective adrenergic agonists. Mannitol and pilocarpine may also be used.

Orbital cellulitis is another ophthalmologic emergency. The eyelids are hot, tender, red, and swollen, and the patient is febrile—but the key finding when the eyelids are pried open is that the pupil is dilated and fixed, and the eye has very limited motion. There is pus in the orbit, and emergency CT scan and drainage have to be done.

Chemical burns of the eye require massive irrigation, like their counterparts elsewhere in the body. Irrigation with plain water has to be started as soon as possible wherever the injury happened; it cannot wait until arrival at the hospital. Once the eye has been pried open and washed under running water for about half an hour, transportation to the ER should be arranged. At the hospital, irrigation with saline is continued, corrosive particles are removed from hidden corners, and before the patient is sent home, pH is tested to assure that no harmful chemicals remain in the conjunctival sac. As is true elsewhere in the body, alkaline burns are worse than acid burns.

Retinal detachment is another emergency that should be recognized by all physicians. The patient reports seeing flashes of light and having "floaters" in the eye. The number of floaters gives a rough idea of the magnitude of the problem. The individual with 1 or 2 floaters may only have vitreous tugging at the retina, with little actual detachment. The person who describes dozens of floaters, or "a snowstorm" within the eye, or a big dark cloud at the top of his visual field has a big horseshoe piece of the retina pulled away and is at risk of ripping out the rest. Emergency intervention, with laser "spot welding," will protect the remaining retina.

Embolic occlusion of the retinal artery is also an emergency, although little can be done about it. The patient (typically elderly) describes sudden loss of vision from one eye. In about 30 minutes the damage will be irreversible, but the standard recommendation is for the patient to breathe into a paper bag and have someone repeatedly press hard on the eye and release while he is in transit to the ER (the idea is to vasodilate and shake the clot into a more distal location, so that a smaller area is ischemic).

Newly diagnosed diabetics need ophthalmologic evaluation if they have type 2, because they may have had it for years before diagnosis was made. Retinal damage may have already occurred, and proper treatment (with the use of lasers) may prevent its progression. Youngsters diagnosed with type 1 are about 20 years away from getting eye problems.

Chapter 10
Otolaryngology (ENT)

Neck Masses

Neck masses can be congenital, inflammatory, or neoplastic. Congenital masses are seen in young people, and typically have been present for years before they become symptomatic (get infected) and medical help is sought. The timetable of inflammatory masses is typically measured in days or weeks. After a few weeks an inflammatory mass has reached some kind of resolution (drained or resolved). The timetable of neoplastic masses is typically several months of relentless growth.

Congenital

Thyroglossal duct cyst is located on the midline, at the level of the hyoid bone, and seems to be somehow connected to the tongue (pulling at the tongue retracts the mass). They are typically 1 or 2 cm in diameter. Surgical removal includes the cyst, the middle segment of the hyoid bone, and the track that leads to the base of the tongue. Some practitioners insist that the location of the normal thyroid should first be ascertained by radionuclide scan.

Branchial cleft cysts occur along the anterior edge of the sternomastoid muscle, anywhere from in front of the tragus to the base of the neck. They are several centimeters in diameter and sometimes have a little opening and blind tract in the skin overlying them.

Cystic hygroma is found at the base of the neck as a large, mushy, ill-defined mass that occupies the entire supraclavicular area and seems to extend deeper into the chest. Indeed, they often extend into the mediastinum, and therefore CT scan before attempted surgical removal is mandatory.

Inflammatory Versus Neoplastic

Most recently discovered enlarged lymph nodes are benign, and therefore an expensive workup should not be undertaken right away. Complete history and physical should be followed by an appointment in 3 to 4 weeks. If the mass is still there, workup then follows.

Persistent enlarged lymph nodes (a history of weeks or months) could still be inflammatory, but neoplasia has to be ruled out. There are several patterns that are suggestive of specific diagnosis, as detailed below.

Lymphoma is typically seen in young people; they often have multiple enlarged nodes (in the neck and elsewhere) and have been suffering from low-grade fever and night sweats. FNA can be done, but usually a node has to be removed for pathologic study to determine specific type. Chemotherapy is the usual treatment.

Metastatic tumor to supraclavicular nodes invariably comes from below the clavicles (and not from the head and neck). Lung or intraabdominal tumors are the usual primaries. The node itself may be removed to help establish a tissue diagnosis.

Squamous cell carcinoma of the mucosae of the head and neck is seen in old men who smoke and drink and have rotten teeth. Patients with AIDS are also prime candidates. Often the first manifestation is a metastatic node in the neck (typically to the jugular chain). The ideal diagnostic workup is a triple endoscopy (or panendoscopy) looking for the primary tumor or tumors. Biopsy of the primary or primaries establishes the diagnosis, and CT scan demonstrates the extent. FNA of the node may be done, but open biopsy of the neck mass should never be performed. An incision in the neck for that purpose will eventually interfere with the appropriate surgical approach for the tumor. Treatment involves resection, radical neck dissection, and very often radiotherapy and platinum-based chemotherapy. Other presentations of squamous cell carcinoma include persistent hoarseness, persistent painless ulcer in the floor of the mouth, and persistent unilateral earache.

Other Tumors

Acoustic nerve neuroma should be suspected in an adult who has sensory hearing loss in one ear, but not the other (and who does not engage in sport shooting that would subject one ear to more noise than the other). MRI is the best diagnostic modality.

Facial nerve tumors produce gradual unilateral facial nerve paralysis affecting both the forehead and the lower face. (Paralysis of sudden onset suggests Bell's palsy.) Gadolinium-enhanced MRI is the best diagnostic study.

Parotid tumors are visible and palpable in front of the ear or around the angle of the mandible. Most are pleomorphic adenomas, which are benign but have potential for malignant degeneration. They do not produce pain or facial nerve paralysis. A hard parotid mass that is painful or has produced paralysis is a parotid cancer. FNA of these tumors may be done, but open biopsy is absolutely contraindicated. A formal superficial parotidectomy (or superficial and deep if the tumor is deep to the facial nerve) is the appropriate way to excise (and thereby biopsy) parotid tumors, preventing recurrences and sparing the facial nerve. Enucleation alone leads to recurrence. In malignant tumors the nerve is sacrificed and a graft done.

Pediatric ENT

Foreign bodies are the cause of unilateral ENT problems in toddlers. A 2-year-old with unilateral earache, unilateral rhinorrhea, or unilateral wheezing has a little toy truck (substitute for your favorite toy if you wish) in his ear canal, up his nose, or into a bronchus. The appropriate endoscopy under anesthesia will allow extraction.

ENT Emergencies and Miscellaneous

Ludwig angina is an abscess of the floor of the mouth, often the result of a bad tooth infection. The usual findings of an abscess are present, but the special issue here is the threat to the airway. Incision and drainage are done, but intubation and tracheostomy may also be needed.

Bell's palsy produces sudden paralysis of the facial nerve for no apparent reason. Although not an emergency per se, current practice includes the use of antiviral medications—and as is the case for other situations in which antivirals are used, prompt and early administration is the key to their success. Steroids are also typically prescribed.

Facial nerve injuries sustained in multiple trauma produce paralysis right away. Patients who have normal nerve function at the time of admission and later develop paralysis have swelling that will resolve spontaneously.

Cavernous sinus thrombosis is heralded by the development of diplopia (from paralysis of extrinsic eye muscles), along with facial pain and high fever, in a patient suffering from frontal or ethmoid sinusitis. This is a rare but very serious emergency (30% mortality) that requires hospitalization. Diagnosis is best done with MRI. Treatment is based on early and aggressive IV antibiotic administration, for a minimum of 3 or 4 weeks, with penicillinase-resistant penicillin plus a third- or fourth-generation cephalosporin. While the cavernous sinus itself would not benefit from operative intervention, the responsible paranasal sinuses should be surgically drained.

Epistaxis in children is typically from nosepicking; the bleeding comes from the anterior septum, and phenylephrine spray and local pressure controls the problem. In an 18-year-old the prime suspects are cocaine abuse (with septal perforation) or juvenile nasopharyngeal angiofibroma. Posterior packing may be needed for the former, and surgical resection is mandatory for the latter (the tumor is benign, but it eats away at nearby structures). In the elderly and hypertensive, nosebleeds can be copious and life-threatening. The blood pressure has to be controlled, and posterior packing is usually required. Sometimes surgical ligation of feeding vessels is the only way to control the problem.

Dizziness may be caused by inner ear disease or cerebral disease. When the inner ear is the culprit, the patients describe the room spinning around them. When the problem is in the brain, the patient is unsteady but the room is perceived to be stable. In the first case meclizine, promethazine, or diazepam may help. In the second case, neurologic workup is in order.

Full-fledged **Ménière disease** includes vertigo, tinnitus, and hearing loss. It is treated primarily with diuretics.

CHAPTER 11
Neurosurgery

Differential Diagnosis Based on Patient History

The timetable and mode of presentation of neurologic disease may provide the first clues as to its nature. Vascular problems have sudden onset, without headache when they are occlusive, and with very severe headache when they are hemorrhagic. Brain tumors have a timetable of months and produce constant, progressive, severe headache, sometimes worse in the mornings. As ICP increases, blurred vision and projectile vomiting are added. If the tumor presses on an area of the brain associated with a particular function, deficits of that function may be evident. Infectious problems have a timetable of days or weeks, and often an identifiable source of infection in the history. Metabolic problems develop rapidly (hours or days) and affect the entire CNS. Degenerative diseases usually have a timetable of years.

Vascular Occlusive Disease

Transient ischemic attacks (TIAs) are sudden, transitory losses of neurologic function that come on without headache and resolve spontaneously leaving no neurologic sequela. The specific symptoms depend on the area of the brain affected, which is in turn related to the vessels involved. The most common origin is high-grade stenosis (70% or above) of the internal carotid, or ulcerated plaque, at the carotid bifurcation. The importance of TIAs is that they are predictors of stroke, and timely elective carotid endarterectomy may prevent or minimize that possibility. Workup starts with noninvasive Duplex studies (high-quality sonogram plus Doppler). Surgery (carotid end-arterectomy) is indicated if the lesions described above are found in the location that explains the neurologic symptoms. Angioplasty and stent can be done if a filter is first deployed to prevent embolization of debris to the brain.

Ischemic stroke also has sudden onset without headache, but the neu-rologic deficits are present for a longer time, leaving permanent sequel-ae. Ischemic strokes that have been present for longer than 3 hours are not amenable to revascularization procedures. An ischemic infarct may be complicated by a hemorrhagic infarct if blood supply to the brain is suddenly increased. Vascular workup will eventually be done to iden-tify lesions that might produce another stroke (and treat them), but for the existing infarct, assessment is by CT scan and therapy is cen-tered on rehabilitation. Treatment of an early ongoing stroke has now become standard practice, with one or more hospitals in each major city equipped with the necessary resources and staff and designated as the places to do it. At the first sign of a sudden-onset neurological defi-cit, the patient is urged to report immediately to the emergency room. CT scan is done first to rule out infarcts that are too extensive to be treated, and to confirm that there is no hemorrhage. If at any time dur-ing this evaluation the neurological functions spontaneously return, the case is reclassified as a TIA and managed accordingly. But if not, no time should be wasted. Intravenous infusion of tissue-type plasmino-gen activator (t-PA) is best if started within 90 minutes, but it can still be done up to 3 hours after the onset of symptoms.

Intracranial Bleeding

Hemorrhagic stroke is seen in the uncontrolled hypertensive who complains of very severe headache of sudden onset and goes on to develop severe neurologic deficits. CT scan is used to evaluate the location and extent of the hemorrhage, and therapy is directed at control of the hypertension and rehabilitation efforts.

Subarachnoid bleeding from intracranial aneurysms has a wide spectrum of severity when it first presents, and some patients are not salvageable—but in many cases a high index of suspicion and a timely diagnosis can be lifesaving. That sort of salvageable patient shows up complaining of extremely severe headache of sudden onset, like no other ever experienced before (a "thunderclap," a headache that is "sudden, severe, and singular"). Because the blood is in the subarachnoid space (there is no hematoma pressing on the brain), there may be no neurologic findings at all, and the patient is sent home. Luckier patients may have meningeal irritation and nuchal rigidity, and be recognized. Those not recognized often return in 10 days with another bleed, perhaps this time a much worse one (the early one is referred to as the "sentinel bleed"). Workup begins with CT scan looking for blood in the subarachnoid space (spinal tap can identify old blood or small amounts of current blood, but it should never be the first test; always start with the CT) and follows with arteriogram to locate the aneurysm (a little devil off the circle of Willis). Clipping is the surgical therapy, and endovascular coiling is the radiological alternative.

Brain Tumors

Most **intracranial tumors** are metastatic, rather than primary, which is not surprising since the brain is one of the four favorite destinations of blood-borne malignant cells—along with bone, liver, and lung. About half come from the lung; the next most common are breast and melanoma. The symptoms are those of a space-occupying lesion (detailed in the next paragraph). A further clinical clue is that the patient has had one of those cancers. About half of primary brain tumors in the adult are gliomas; meningiomas account for about 20%. The most malignant intracranial tumor is glioblastoma multiforme, a type of glioma. Meningiomas are usually benign. The treatment of brain tumors is typically multimodal, including surgery, radiation, and chemotherapy for those cases where the blood-brain barrier has already been breached.

Brain tumors may offer no clue as to location if they press on a "silent area" of the brain. The only history will be progressively increasing headache for several months, worse in the mornings, and eventually accompanied by signs of increased ICP: blurred vision, papilledema, projectile vomiting—and at the extreme of the spectrum, bradycardia and hypertension (due to the Cushing reflex). Brain tumors can be visualized very well on CT scan, but MRI gives better detail and is the preferred study. While awaiting surgical removal, increased ICP is treated with high-dose steroids (i.e., dexamethasone [trade name Decadron]).

Clinical localization of brain tumors may be possible by virtue of specific neurologic deficits or symptom patterns. For example, the motor strip and speech centers are often affected in tumors that press on the lateral side of the brain, producing symptoms on the opposite side of the body (people speak with the same side of the brain that controls their dominant hand). Other classic clinical pictures include the following:

Tumors at the base of the frontal lobe produce inappropriate behavior, optic nerve atrophy on the side of the tumor, papilledema on the other side, and anosmia (Foster-Kennedy syndrome).

Craniopharyngioma occurs in youngsters who are short for their age, and they show bitemporal hemianopsia and a calcified lesion above the sella on CT scan.

Prolactinomas produce amenorrhea and galactorrhea in young women. Diagnostic workup includes ruling out pregnancy (pregnancy test), ruling out hypothyroidism (TSH), determination of prolactin level, and MRI of the sella. Therapy with bromocriptine, or a similar drug, is used in most cases. Transnasal, trans-sphenoidal surgical removal is reserved for those who wish to get pregnant or those who fail to respond to bromocriptine.

Acromegaly is recognized by the huge hands, feet, tongue, and jaws (and in the USMLE exam by the picture of a man showing both hands on either side of his face in the frontal view, and a long prominent jaw in the lateral view). Additionally, there is hypertension, diabetes, sweaty hands, headache, and a history of wedding bands or hats that no longer fit. Workup starts with determination of somatomedin C, and pituitary MRI. Surgical removal is preferred (transnasal or trans-sphenoidal) but radiation is an option. The somatic changes are irreversible.

Pituitary apoplexy occurs when there is bleeding into a pituitary tumor, with subsequent destruction of the pituitary gland. The history may have clues to the long-standing presence of the pituitary tumor (headache, visual loss, endocrine problems), and the acute episode starts with a severe headache followed by signs of increased compression of nearby structures by the hematoma (deterioration of remaining vision, bilateral pallor of the optic nerves) and pituitary destruction (stupor and hypotension). Steroid replacement is urgently needed, and eventually other hormones will need to be replaced. MRI or CT scan will show the extent of the problem.

Tumors of the pineal gland produce loss of upper gaze and the physical finding known as "sunset eyes" (Parinaud syndrome).

Brain tumors in children are usually in the posterior fossa. Medulloblastoma is the most common type. It arises in the cerebellum and gives the classic cerebellar symptoms, such as stumbling around and truncal ataxia. The second most common type is ependymoma. Some of those pivot on a pedicle, and affected children often assume the knee-chest position to open the flow of cerebrospinal fluid and relieve their headache.

Brain abscess shows many of the same manifestations of brain tumors (it is a space-occupying lesion), but a much shorter timetable (a week or two). There is fever, and usually an obvious source of the infection nearby, like otitis media and mastoiditis. They have a very typical appearance on CT, thus the more expensive MRI is not needed. Actual resection is required.

Pain Syndromes

Trigeminal neuralgia (tic douloureux) produces extremely severe, sharp shooting pain "like a bolt of lightning" in the face, brought about by touching a specific area and lasting about 60 seconds. Patients are in their 60s and have a completely normal neurologic exam. The only finding on physical may be an unshaven area in the face (the trigger zone, which the patient avoids touching). MRI is done to rule out organic lesions. Treatment with anticonvulsants is often successful (notably carbamazapine). If not, radiofrequency ablation can be done. Some surgeons believe pounding from a nearby vessel may be responsible, and they advocate an operation to separate them.

Reflex sympathetic dystrophy (causalgia) develops several months after a crushing injury. There is constant, burning, agonizing pain that does not respond to the usual analgesics. The pain is aggravated by the slightest stimulation of the area. The extremity is cold, cyanotic, and moist. A successful sympathetic block is diagnostic, and surgical sympathectomy is curative.

Chapter 12
Urology

Urologic Emergencies

Testicular torsion is seen in young adolescents. They have very severe testicular pain of sudden onset, but no fever, pyuria, or history of recent mumps. The testis is swollen, exquisitely tender, "high riding," and with a "horizontal lie." The cord is not tender. This is one of the few urologic emergencies, and time wasted doing any tests is tantamount to malpractice. Immediate surgical intervention is indicated. After the testis is untwisted, an orchiopexy is done. Many urologists also fix the other side.

Acute epididymitis is the condition with which testicular torsion could be confused. It happens in young men old enough to be sexually active, and it also starts with severe testicular pain of sudden onset. There is fever and pyuria, and the testis although swollen and very tender is in the normal position. The cord is also very tender. Lifting the scrotum helps. Acute epididymitis is treated with antibiotics, but the possibility of missing a diagnosis of testicular torsion is so dreadful that sonogram is done to rule it out.

The combination of obstruction and infection of the urinary tract is the other condition (besides testicular torsion) that is a dire emergency. Any situation in which these 2 conditions coexist can lead to destruction of the kidney in a few hours, and potentially to death from sepsis. A typical scenario is a patient who is being allowed to pass a ureteral stone spontaneously and who suddenly develops chills, fever spike (104° or 105°F), and flank pain. In addition to IV antibiotics, immediate decompression of the urinary tract above the obstruction is required. This is accomplished by the quickest and simplest means (in this example, ureteral stent or percutaneous nephrostomy), deferring more elaborate instrumentations for a later, safer date.

An erection lasting more than 4 hours after the use of erectile dysfunction drugs is also a dire emergency. The TV ads say so. But they gloss over the treatment. It may be necessary to stick needles into that erect penis, to draw out blood. Marketing strategy suggests it's best not to mention that.

Urinary tract infection (cystitis) is very common in women of reproductive age, and it requires no elaborate workup. They have frequency, painful urination, with small volumes of cloudy and malodorous urine. Empiric antimicrobial therapy is used. More serious infections, like pyelonephritis, or any urinary tract infection in children or young men requires urinary cultures and some kind of a "urologic workup" to rule out concomitant obstruction as the reason for the serious infection.

Urologic workup uses 3 tests: sonogram, CT scan, and/or cystoscopy. The first is indicated for dilation and obstruction; the second is ideal for renal tumors; and the third is the only way to detect early bladder cancers. The old intravenous pyelogram (IVP) has almost disappeared, along with the nephrotoxicity and allergic reactions that made it risky.

Pyelonephritis produces chills, high fever, nausea and vomiting, and flank pain. Hospitalization, IV antibiotics (guided by cultures), and urologic workup (CT or sonogram) are required.

Acute bacterial prostatitis is seen in older men who have chills, fever, dysuria, urinary frequency, diffuse low back pain, and an exquisitely tender prostate on rectal exam. IV antibiotics are indicated, and care should be taken not to repeat any more rectal exams. Continued prostatic massage could lead to septic shock.

Congenital Urologic Disease

Posterior urethral valves are the most common reason for a newborn boy not to urinate during the first day of life (meatal stenosis should also be looked for). Catheterization can be done to empty the bladder (the valves will not present an obstacle to the catheter). Voiding cystourethrogram is the diagnostic test, and endoscopic fulguration or resection will get rid of them.

Hypospadias is easily noted on physical exam. The urethral opening is on the ventral side of the penis, somewhere between the tip and the base of the shaft. Circumcision should never be done on such a child, inasmuch as the skin of the prepuce will be needed for the plastic reconstruction that will eventually be done.

Urinary tract infection in children should always lead to a urologic workup. The cause may be vesicoureteral reflux or some other congenital anomaly.

Vesicoureteral reflux and infection produce burning on urination, frequency, low abdominal and perineal pain, flank pain, and fever and chills in a child. Start treatment of the infection (with empiric antibiotics first, followed by culture-guided choice), and do voiding cystourethrogram looking for the reflux. If found, long-term antibiotics are used until the child "grows out of the problem."

Low implantation of a ureter is usually asymptomatic in little boys but leads to a fascinating clinical presentation in little girls. The patient feels normally the need to void, and voids normally at appropriate intervals (urine deposited into the bladder by the normal ureter), but she is also wet with urine all the time (urine that drips into the vagina from the low-implanted ureter). Careful vaginoscopy should identify the ectopic ureter. IVPs are best avoided in children. Corrective surgery will follow.

Ureteropelvic junction (UPJ) obstruction can also produce a fascinating clinical presentation. The anomaly at the UPJ allows normal urinary output to flow without difficulty, but if a large diuresis occurs, the narrow area cannot handle it. Thus the classic presentation is an adolescent who goes on a beer-drinking binge for the first time in his life and develops colicky flank pain.

Tumors

Hematuria is the most common presentation for cancers of the kidney, ureter, or bladder. Actually most cases of hematuria are caused by benign disease, but except for the adult who has a trace of urine after significant trauma, any patient presenting with hematuria needs a workup to rule out cancer.

The workup of hematuria begins with CT scan and continues with cystoscopy, which is the only reliable way to rule out cancer of the bladder.

Renal cell carcinoma in its full-blown picture produces hematuria, flank pain, and a flank mass. They can also produce hypercalcemia, erythrocytosis, and elevated liver enzymes. That full-blown picture is rarely seen nowadays, when most patients are worked up as soon as they have hematuria. CT gives the best detail, showing the mass to be heterogenic solid tumor (and alerting the urologist to potential growth into the renal vein and the vena cava, which could become a lethal pulmonary embolus if dislodged during the nephrectomy). Surgery is the only effective therapy. Targeted chemo is under investigation.

Cancer of the bladder (transitional cell cancer in most cases) has a very close correlation with smoking (even more so than cancer of the lung) and usually presents with hematuria. Sometimes there are irritative voiding symptoms, and patients may have been treated for urinary tract infection even though cultures were negative and they were afebrile. Although cystoscopy is the best way to diagnose these, it should be preceded by CT scan. Both surgery and intravesical BCG have therapeutic roles, and a very high rate of local recurrence makes lifelong close follow-up a necessity.

Prostatic cancer incidence increases with age. Most are asymptomatic and have to be sought by rectal exam (rock-hard discrete nodule) and prostatic specific antigen (PSA; elevated levels for age group). Transrectal needle biopsy (guided by sonogram when discovered by PSA) establishes diagnosis. CT helps assess extent and choose therapy. Surgery and/or radiation are choices. Widespread bone metastases respond for a few years to androgen ablation, surgical (orchiectomy) or medical (luteinizing hormone-releasing hormone agonists, or antiandrogens like flutamide).

Testicular cancer affects young men, in whom it presents as a painless testicular mass. Because benign testicular tumors are virtually nonexistent, biopsy is done with a radical orchiectomy by the inguinal route. Blood samples are taken pre-op for serum markers (α-fetoprotein and β-human chorionic gonadotropin [β-hCG]), which will be useful for follow-up. Further surgery for lymph node dissection may be done in some cases. Most testicular cancers are exquisitely radiosensitive and chemosensitive (platinum-based chemotherapy), offering many options for successful treatment in advanced, metastatic disease.

Retention and Incontinence

Acute urinary retention is seen very commonly in men who already have significant symptoms from benign prostatic hypertrophy. It is often precipitated during a cold, by the use of antihistamines and nasal drops, and by abundant fluid intake. The patient wants to void but cannot, and the huge distended bladder is palpable. An indwelling bladder catheter needs to be placed and left in for at least 3 days. First line of long-term therapy is alpha-blockers, the most selective of which is tamsulosin. 5-Alpha-reductase inhibitors, like finasteride or dutasteride, are used for very large glands (more than 40 g). Minimally invasive procedures using thermal ablation of prostatic tissue have not gained popularity. The traditional transurethral resection of the prostate (TURP), although rarely done, remains the final surgical option for benign prostatic hypertrophy.

Postoperative urinary retention is also very common, and sometimes it masquerades as incontinence. The patient may not feel the need to void because of post-op pain, medications, etc., but will report that every few minutes there is involuntary release of small amounts of urine. A huge distended bladder will be palpable, confirming that the problem is overflow incontinence from retention. Indwelling bladder catheter is needed.

Stress incontinence is also very common. It is seen in middle-age women who have had many pregnancies and vaginal deliveries. They leak small amounts of urine whenever intraabdominal pressure suddenly increases. This includes sneezing, laughing, getting out of a chair, or lifting a heavy object. They do not have any incontinence during the night. Examination will show a weak pelvic floor, with the prolapsed bladder neck outside of the "high-pressure" abdominal area. Surgical repair of the pelvic floor is indicated in advanced cases with large cystoceles. Pelvic floor exercises may be sufficient for early cases.

Stones

Passage of ureteral stones produces the classic colicky flank pain, with irradiation to the inner thigh and labia or scrotum, and sometimes nausea and vomiting. Most stones are visible in CT scan. Although there is an impressive array of fancy gadgetry available to deal with urinary stones, intervention is not always needed. Small (3 mm or less) stones at the ureterovesical junction have a 70% chance of passing spontaneously. Such cases can be handled with analgesics, plenty of fluids, and watchful waiting. On the other hand, a 7-mm stone at the UPJ only has a 5% probability of passing.

Intervention will be required. The most common tool used is extra-corporeal shock-wave lithotripsy (ESWL). Sometimes ESWL cannot be used (pregnant women, bleeding diathesis, stones that are several centimeters large). Other options include basket extraction, sonic probes, laser beams, and open surgery. Although there is specific therapy for the prevention of recurrences in defined types of stones, abundant water intake is universally applicable.

Miscellaneous

Pneumaturia is almost always caused by fistulization between the bladder and the GI tract, most commonly the sigmoid colon, and most commonly from diverticulitis (second possibility is cancer of the sigmoid, and cancer of the bladder is a very distant third). Workup starts with CT scan, which will show the inflammatory diverticular mass. Sigmoidoscopy is needed later to rule out cancer. Surgical therapy is required.

Impotence can be organic or psychogenic. Psychogenic impotence has sudden onset, is partner- or situation-specific, does not interfere with nocturnal erections (which can be tested with a strip of perforated postage stamps), and can be effectively treated with psychotherapy only if it is done promptly. Organic impotence, if caused by trauma, will also have sudden onset, specifically related to the traumatic event (after pelvic surgery, because of nerve damage, or after trauma to the perineum, which involves arterial disruption). Organic impotence because of chronic disease (arteriosclerosis, diabetes) has very gradual onset, going from erections not lasting long enough, to being of poor quality, to not happening at all (including absence of nocturnal erections). Sildenafil, tadalafil, and vardenafil have become obvious first choices of therapy in many cases, but there are many other options, including vascular surgery (well suited for those with arterial injury), suction devices (that can be used on almost everybody), and prosthetic implants (which are irreversible and fraught with complications).

Diagnosing Nocturnal Erections with Postage Stamps: A Generation Gap

Some students have been puzzled by the reference to the use of a roll of postage stamps to test for nocturnal erections. This is because the only postage stamps they have ever seen come in little booklets, from where they are peeled away to be affixed to an envelope.

Older physicians remember the rolls of paper stamps that had rows of perforations between them and had to be licked or dampened with a sponge to glue them into place. To test for nocturnal erections, those physicians would wrap a circumference of stamps around the shaft of the patient's flaccid penis and glue them into position just below the glans. The patient slept with this device in place. If the ring of stamps was intact in the morning, there had been no nocturnal erections. If it was torn along the perforations, we assumed the penis had been engorged.

Now you know.

CHAPTER 13
Bariatric Surgery

The most pressing current public health problem in the United States is a galloping epidemic of obesity. The statistics are frightening. Nuclear war or global warming may not be what brings our doomsday; we are literally eating ourselves to death. Super-obese individuals (those with BMI over 40) are dying from diabetes, sleep apnea, heart disease, and other complications of their enormous size.

We need a breakthrough to recalibrate the neurological centers that produce hunger and satiety. But we have not yet discovered it, and these patients cannot wait for us to figure it out. By necessity, then, we are addressing the problem of morbid obesity by messing up patients' perfectly normal gastrointestinal tracts with bariatric surgery.

I cannot tell you what is the best way to modify the gut. Every single operation that has been devised to promote weight loss has ultimately been discarded owing to its excessive complications. The best I can do is to give you a suitable example, which uses a technical trick that surgeons often resort to when rearranging the GI tract.

A current favorite is called the Roux-en-Y gastric bypass. This procedure creates a small gastric pouch by dividing and stapling the body of the stomach.

That small reservoir is eventually connected to the small bowel, while most of the remaining stomach and the entire duodenum are bypassed. The area would look like this:

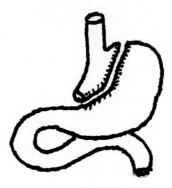

The next step is to bring up a loop of small bowel to join that tiny gastric pouch, as depicted in the second drawing. While this arrangement allows food into the bowel, it also permits gastric juice, bile, and pancreatic fluid to flow into the pouch and nearby esophagus, eroding these structures. Not good. We need a one-way connection.

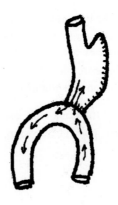

Enter Dr. Cesar Roux, a Swiss surgeon who devised the procedure now named for him. Instead of creating a direct anastomosis, Roux-en-Y gastric bypass divides the small bowel, brings up the distal segment where needed, and reconnects the upper part about 30 cm lower down. Unidirectional peristaltic flow prevents the undesirable reflux. The resulting shape looks like the letter "Y," thus the name of the operation.

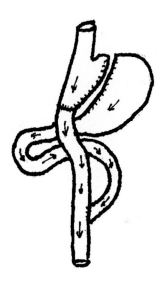

Chapter 14
Organ Transplantation

Selection of donors has been liberalized tremendously to help alleviate the acute shortage of organs. Virtually all brain-dead patients are potential candidates, regardless of age. Donors with specific infections (like hepatitis or HIV) can be used for recipients who have the same disease. Even donors with metastatic cancer can donate corneas. The general rule for regular physicians is that all potential donors are referred to the harvesting teams, and they will exclude the few that cannot be used at all.

Transplant rejection can happen in 3 ways: hyperacute, acute, and chronic rejection.

Hyperacute rejection is a vascular thrombosis that occurs within minutes of reestablishing blood supply to the organ. It is caused by preformed antibodies. It is prevented by ABO matching and lymphocytotoxic crossmatch, and thus it is not seen clinically.

Acute rejection occurs after the first 5 days, and usually within the first 3 months. Episodes occur even though the patient is on maintenance immunosuppression. Current maintenance protocols include tacrolimus and mycophenolate mofetil, with or without prednisone. Signs of organ dysfunction suggest acute rejection, and biopsy confirms it. In the case of the liver, technical problems are more commonly encountered than immunologic rejection. Thus the first order of business when liver function deteriorates after a transplant (rising γ-glutamyltransferase [GGT], alkaline phosphatase, and bilirubin) is to rule out biliary obstruction by ultrasound and vascular thrombosis by Doppler. In the case of the heart, signs of functional deterioration occur too late to allow effective therapy, thus routine ventricular biopsies (by way of the jugular, superior vena cava, and right atrium) are done at set intervals. The first line of therapy for acute rejection is steroid boluses. If unsuccessful, antilymphocyte agents (OKT3) have been used, but their high toxicity is a problem. Newer antithymocyte serum is tolerated better.

Chronic rejection is seen years after the transplant, with gradual, insidious loss of organ function. It is poorly understood and irreversible. Although we have no treatment for it, patients suspected of having it have the transplant biopsied in the hope that it may be a delayed (and treatable) case of acute rejection.

Section II
Practice Questions

Questions

This section provides 180 multiple-choice practice questions for your ongoing self-assessment. They contain only the key combination of facts that should be immediately recognized by an astute clinician.

For each practice question, the answer key on pages 243–250 indicates both the correct answer choice and the location in Section I: Surgery Review where the relevant explanatory information can be found. If you have carefully read the text, the correct answer for most of the practice questions will be obvious to you. Where you need to reinforce your knowledge, the page and paragraph references in the answer key will direct you to what needs to be read again.

1. A 27-year-old man is stabbed in the right chest with a 5-cm-long knife blade. On arrival at the ER he is wide awake and alert, speaking with a normal tone of voice, but complaining of moderate shortness of breath. He has no breath sounds over his right hemithorax, but the rest of the initial survey is negative. Pulse oximetry shows a saturation of 85. Management of his airway at this time requires which of the following?

   A. Airway does not need to be secured at this time.

   B. Awake orotracheal intubation.

   C. Blind nasotracheal intubation.

   D. Cricothyroidotomy.

   E. Orotracheal intubation with short-acting anesthetic induction.

2. A 53-year-old man is placed on warfarin after a sigmoid resection for cancer. His prothrombin time becomes quite high, but he has no overt signs of bleeding, so the clinical team decides not to reverse his anticoagulation with vitamin K. A couple of hours later he complains of back pain. A portable x-ray of his lumbar spine is noncontributory. Two hours after that, he goes into shock. EKG and troponins are normal, and it is assumed he has developed septic shock. Initial treatment with antibiotics and a steroid bolus produces dramatic restoration of normal vital signs. However, 2 hours after that he is back in shock, deteriorates rapidly, and dies. An autopsy is likely to reveal that he:

   A. Bled into and destroyed his adrenal glands.

   B. Extruded a lumbar disk at L4–L5.

   C. Had a massive myocardial infarction.

   D. Had very extensive bilateral pulmonary emboli.

   E. Leaked 3 liters of blood from an aortic aneurysm into his retroperitoneal space.

3. During a school picnic, a 33-year-old teacher accidentally bumps into a beehive and is repeatedly stung by angry bees. On arrival at the ER her blood pressure is 72 over 20 and her pulse rate is 150, but she looks warm and flushed rather than pale and cold. Her CVP is low. The reason for the low blood pressure reading is:

   A. Cardiogenic shock.

   B. Hypovolemia.

   C. Massive vasoconstriction.

   D. Pain and fright.

   E. Vasomotor shock.

4. During an attempted robbery, an 18-year-old man is hit over the head with a blunt instrument. He manages to escape further injuries, and he comes to a nearby ER with all his family in tow because it hurts where he got hit. He is completely lucid, was never unconscious, and can remember all the details of his ordeal. A CT scan of his head shows a linear skull fracture. There is no scalp wound over that area, and there are no intracranial hematomas. Further management should include which of the following?

   A. Closely monitor blood pressure for possible development of hypovolemic shock.

   B. Initiate exploratory craniotomy to assess intracranial injuries.

   C. Expose the fracture in the OR to be repaired with plates and screws.

   D. Repeat the CT scan, this time including the entire neck.

   E. Send the man home to the care of his family.

5. A 54-year-old man involved in a high-speed, head-on automobile collision is in coma. Both of his pupils are dilated and fixed. CT scan shows a small, semilunar, crescent-shaped intracranial hematoma hugging the inside of the skull. There is no deviation of his midline structures. What would help this patient the most would be:

   A. High-dose steroids.

   B. Monitoring of intracranial pressure.

   C. Prompt surgical evacuation of his epidural hematoma.

   D. Prompt surgical evacuation of his subdural hematoma.

   E. Systemic vasodilators and alpha-blockers.

n engage in a knife fight, in which one of them is dly stabbed. One of the wounds is deep in his back, just right of the midline. Distal to that injury, he has paralysis and loss of proprioception on the right side, and loss of pain perception on the left side. The diagnosis is:

A. Anterior cord syndrome.

B. Central cord syndrome.

C. Complete transection of the spinal cord.

D. Hemisection of the spinal cord (Brown-Séquard).

E. Posterior cord syndrome.

7. In the course of a mugging, a 72-year-old man is repeatedly struck in the chest with a baseball bat. X-rays show a fracture of the right fifth rib at the level of the midclavicular line. This injury is best treated by:

A. Binding of the chest wall to limit motion.

B. Enough systemic analgesics to depress his respiratory drive.

C. Intercostal nerve block and analgesia by epidural catheter.

D. Open reduction and internal fixation.

E. Supplemental oxygen by endotracheal tube.

8. In an automobile accident, a 55-year-old man sustains several rib fractures. At the time of admission, his lungs are clear on x-rays and blood gases are normal. Two days later the lungs "white out" and he has hypoxemia and hypercapnia. The most likely diagnosis is:

   A. Adult respiratory distress syndrome (ARDS).

   B. Fat embolism.

   C. Pulmonary contusion.

   D. Pulmonary embolism.

   E. Tension pneumothorax.

9. A 27-year-old police officer is shot in the abdomen at close range with a .45-caliber revolver. The entrance wound is just to the left of the umbilicus, and the bullet is seen in x-rays to be embedded in the right psoas muscle. He is hemodynamically stable, and the abdomen is moderately tender to palpation. Assessment of the extent of his intraabdominal injuries will best be made by:

   A. CT scan of the abdomen.

   B. Close clinical observation.

   C. Diagnostic peritoneal lavage.

   D. Exploratory laparotomy.

   E. Sonogram done in the ER.

10. After receiving 10 units of packed red cells during surgery for massive intraabdominal injuries sustained in a car accident, a 29-year-old man is noted to be oozing blood from all dissected raw surfaces, as well as his IV line sites. His core temperature is normal. The next step in management should be:

    A. Abort the operation, pack the abdomen, and close it tight.

    B. Emergency coagulation profile and specific therapy.

    C. Empiric administration of fresh frozen plasma and platelet packs.

    D. Empiric administration of vitamin K.

    E. Proceed with surgery and give additional banked blood as needed.

11. In the evaluation of a 23-year-old man with a pelvic fracture sustained in a severe car accident, it is noted that he has blood at the meatus and a scrotal hematoma. His urological workup should begin with:

    A. Cystoscopy.

    B. Intravenous pyelogram (IVP).

    C. Retrograde cystogram via Foley catheter.

    D. Retrograde urethrogram.

    E. Scrotal sonogram.

12. An 18-year-old male is shot point-blank with a .38-caliber revolver. The entrance wound is in the anterior, lateral aspect of his upper thigh, and the bullet is embedded in the muscles posterolateral to his intact femur. The entry wound is carefully cleaned in the ER. What else does he need?

    A. Arteriogram.

    B. Doppler studies.

    C. Surgical exploration of the femoral vessels.

    D. Surgical removal of the bullet.

    E. Tetanus prophylaxis.

13. A 33-year-old woman shows up with a full-thickness, circumferential burn in her upper arm, sustained when her shirt caught fire as she was roasting marshmallows at a picnic. She will need compulsive monitoring of:

    A. Blood gases.

    B. Body weight.

    C. Carboxyhemoglobin levels.

    D. Myoglobinemia and myoglobinuria.

    E. Peripheral pulses and capillary filling.

14. A 33-year-old woman seeks immediate medical attention for a severe burn that she accidentally suffered. A hot iron fell on her lap when she was pressing the laundry. The shape and size of the iron are clearly delineated on her thigh, and the small area is clearly a full-thickness, fresh, clean third-degree burn. She would be an ideal candidate to be treated with:

    A. Application of mafenide acetate.

    B. Application of silver sulfadiazine.

    C. Immediate excision and grafting.

    D. Repeated debridements and wet-to-dry dressings.

    E. Use of triple antibiotic ointment.

15. A newborn baby has uneven gluteal folds, and during physical examination his right hip can be dislocated and put back in place. An older sibling had the same problem, for which he wore a Pavlik harness for 6 months. This child has:

    A. Developmental dysphasia of the hip.

    B. Congenital absence of the femoral head.

    C. Legg-Calvé-Perthes disease (avascular necrosis).

    D. Septic hip.

    E. Slipped capital femoral epiphysis.

16. A 4-year-old child falls down the stairs and fractures the mid-shaft of his humerus. The fracture is easily reduced and placed in a cast at an urgent care clinic. When seen by his pediatrician 2 days later, he seems to be doing fine, but AP and lateral x-rays show significant angulation of the broken bone. You can expect that this child will:

    A. Develop uneven growth due to damage of the growth plate.

    B. Have permanent deformity, but compensate by redirecting bone growth.

    C. Have permanent deformity unless the fracture is reset.

    D. Remodel the fracture and have no permanent deformity.

    E. Require open reduction and internal fixation.

17. A 22-year-old man had a motorcycle accident in which he sustained several bilateral femur fractures. He is currently in the ICU with respiratory failure presumed to be due to fat embolism, being treated on a respirator. He had been fully conscious throughout but has suddenly gone into coma. An MRI of the brain shows a "star-field pattern." This new development suggests that:

    A. A subdural hematoma has developed.

    B. Fat droplets have reached the brain.

    C. He now has irreversible traumatic brain damage.

    D. Pulmonary failure has led to anoxia of the central nervous system.

    E. The respirator has inadvertently produced an air embolism.

18. A 78-year-old man is brought in from his nursing home, where he had fallen. As he lies on the stretcher, his right leg appears shortened and externally rotated. X-rays demonstrate an intertrochanteric fracture of his right hip. The best treatment would be:

    A. Open reduction, internal fixation, and post-op anticoagulation.

    B. Open reduction, internal fixation, and post-op clot busters.

    C. Removal of the femoral head and replacement with a prosthesis.

    D. Skeletal traction and vena cava filter.

    E. Total hip replacement.

19. A fracture of the tibia and fibula has been treated by closed reduction and casting. The patient complains of increasing pain, so the cast is removed 6 hours later to allow examination of the leg. The calf muscles feel tight, and the patient has excruciating pain when the toes are passively extended. This patient will need:

    A. Arteriogram.

    B. Fasciotomy.

    C. Nerve block prior to recasting.

    D. Open reduction and internal fixation.

    E. Recasting with a looser cast.

20. While repairing an elevator shaft, a 39-year-old worker falls from a height of 2 stories, landing on his feet. Both calcanei are obviously fractured. Further evaluation should include:

    A. X-rays of the femur.

    B. X-rays of the knee.

    C. X-rays of the lower leg.

    D. X-rays of the pelvis.

    E. X-rays of thoracic and lumbar spine.

21. An unbelted 23-year-old driver loses control of his convertible during an evening drive. He is ejected as the vehicle falls into a wooded ravine, and he sustains multiple soft tissue wounds as he plunges through the trees. The man is reported missing and is rescued the following morning. At the hospital it is determined that he has no internal injuries, but he spends several hours in the operating room having his wounds cleaned, irrigated, and debrided. Which of the following would be most helpful to prevent infections from developing afterward?

    A. Constant, low positive air pressure applied to the wounds by mechanical devices.

    B. Hermetically sealing the sutured wounds to prevent contact with the air.

    C. Infusing intravenous metronidazole for the next 5 days.

    D. Leaving the skin and subcutaneous tissue open until granulation tissue covers the latter.

    E. Splinting the extremities where there are soft tissue wounds.

22. A 52-year-old man has an indolent, dirty-looking ulcer with heaped-up tissue edges, located over the dorsum of his right foot. He says he has had an ulcer there for at least 30 years, following an untreated third-degree burn that healed by itself. He had not been concerned, because that injury has broken down and healed many times over the years, but now it looks "different" and it is getting larger. The diagnosis is most likely to be provided by:

    A. Arteriograms.

    B. Biopsy of the ulcer edge.

    C. Cultures of the ulcer base.

    D. Doppler studies.

    E. Venous pressure tracings.

23. An elderly man needs palliative surgery for a cancer of the esophagus. He has lost 20% of his body weight over the past 2 months, and his serum albumin is 2.7. Further testing reveals anergy to injected skin-test antigens and a serum transferrin level of less than 200 mg/dL. His operative risk is:

    A. Excellent because he shows sign of adaptation to starvation.

    B. Only slightly worse than average.

    C. Prohibitive and not amenable to short-term interventions.

    D. Very high, but amenable to correction if TPN is used and feeding in the gut is avoided.

    E. Very high, but could be improved considerably with 7–10 days of intensive nutritional support delivered to his gut.

24. A 69-year-old man had a right hemicolectomy yesterday. He reports severe, constricting retrosternal pain of sudden onset, radiating to his left arm. He is tachycardic, sweating profusely, and very anxious. The diagnosis is most likely to be revealed by:

    A. Blood gases.

    B. Chest x-ray.

    C. EKG and troponins.

    D. Spiral CT scan.

    E. Ventilation-perfusion scan.

25. A cirrhotic patient goes into coma after performance of an emergency portacaval shunt for bleeding esophageal varices. The laboratory test most likely to reveal the reason for the neurological deterioration is:

    A. Blood alcohol levels.

    B. Blood gases.

    C. Blood sugar.

    D. Serum ammonium.

    E. Serum sodium.

26. A 62-year-old man is recovering from a subtotal gastrectomy for gastric cancer with a gastroduodenal anastomosis. A Penrose drain has been left in the area. On the sixth postoperative day he began to drain about 2 liters per day of green fluid. He has no abdominal pain, fever, or signs of peritoneal irritation. At this time his management should be:

A. Emergency reclosure of his abdominal incision.

B. Fluid replacement, nutritional support, and protection of the abdominal wall.

C. Fluid restriction and oral intake of mostly solid foods.

D. Intensive medical management with H2 blockers and proton pump inhibitors.

E. Surgical closure of the fistula after antibiotic bowel prep.

27. A patient with severe peptic ulcer disease develops pyloric obstruction, and he has protracted vomiting of clear gastric contents (without blood or bile) for several days. He looks clinically dehydrated, and his serum electrolytes show sodium of 134, chloride 82, potassium 2.9, and bicarbonate 34 (all in mEq/L). Rehydration would best be accomplished with:

A. Dextrose 5% in water (D5W).

B. Half-normal saline with added sodium bicarbonate.

C. Half-normal saline with added sodium lactate.

D. Normal saline with added KCl.

E. Ringer lactate.

28. A 62-year-old woman has been having heartburn for several years, and from time to time she complains of epigastric pain that is relieved with over-the-counter antacid medications. In the last few months her pain has been almost constant and no longer responds to self-medication. The evaluation of her problem will best be done with:

    A. Barium swallow.

    B. Esophageal manometry.

    C. Gastrografin swallow.

    D. pH monitoring.

    E. Upper GI endoscopy.

29. For the past 5 days, a 53-year-old man has been having colicky abdominal pain, protracted vomiting, and progressive abdominal distension. His last bowel movement was 3 days ago, and he is not passing any gas per rectum. On physical exam he has high-pitched bowel sounds but no signs of peritoneal irritation. He has a well-healed midline scar from an exploratory laparotomy for a gunshot wound done 4 years ago. X-rays show dilated loops of small bowel with air-fluid levels. At this time the best management would be:

    A. Antibiotics, anticholinergics, and gentle laxatives.

    B. H2 blockers, antacids, and gastric lavage.

    C. NPO, nasogastric suction, IV fluids, and careful observation.

    D. Rectal tube and colonic irrigation.

    E. Surgical intervention within the next hour.

30. A 61-year-old man reports bright red blood on the toilet paper after evacuation. Arrangements are made to do digital rectal exam, anoscopy, and proctosigmoidoscopy. Most likely the source of his bleeding will be found to be:

    A. Anal fissure.

    B. Anal prolapse.

    C. External hemorrhoids.

    D. Fistula-in-ano.

    E. Internal hemorrhoids.

31. A 68-year-old man has had 3 large bowel movements that he describes as made up entirely of dark red blood. The last one was 20 minutes ago. He is diaphoretic and pale, with a blood pressure of 90 over 70 and pulse rate of 110. Inspection of his mouth and nose shows no blood or lesions that might have bled recently. A nasogastric tube is inserted, and aspiration returns clear green fluid without blood. The source of his bleeding is:

    A. Between the ligament of Treitz and the ileocecal valve.

    B. Distal to the ligament of Treitz.

    C. Distal to the pylorus.

    D. Proximal to the ileocecal valve.

    E. Proximal to the ligament of Treitz.

32. A 49-year-old, obese woman presents with abdominal pain. She has a history of 3 prior episodes of left lower-quadrant abdominal pain, for which she was briefly hospitalized and treated with antibiotics. She began to feel discomfort 12 hours ago, and now she has constant left lower-quadrant pain, tenderness, and a vaguely palpable mass in the left lower-quadrant of the abdomen. She has fever and leukocytosis, and a pelvic exam is negative for OB-GYN pathology. The next diagnostic study indicated in this patient is:

    A. Abdominal sonogram.

    B. Barium enema.

    C. CT scan of the abdomen.

    D. Colonoscopy.

    E. Exploratory laparotomy.

33. A 39-year-old woman has increasing jaundice, first noted 3 weeks ago. Her physical exam is otherwise unremarkable. Her current laboratory values show a total bilirubin of 18, of which 12 is conjugated. There is minimal elevation of transaminases, and alkaline phosphatase is 4 times higher than the lab's reference normal value. The next diagnostic study should be:

    A. Abdominal sonogram of the right upper quadrant.

    B. Endoscopic retrograde cholangiopancreatography (ERCP).

    C. Percutaneous liver biopsy.

    D. Red cell fragility tests.

    E. Serology titers for hepatitis.

34. A 47-year-old alcoholic man is having epigastric and midab-dominal pain, which began shortly after he ate a large meal. The pain reached maximum intensity in about 12 hours and is now constant, severe, and radiating to his back. He vomited early on and has continued to retch even after his stomach was empty. Although he has discomfort when his upper abdomen is palpated, the physical exam is less impressive than the severity of his pain would suggest. He is afebrile. Serum lipase is very elevated, and hematocrit is 54. The most likely diagnosis is:

    A. Acute cholecystitis.

    B. Acute edematous pancreatitis.

    C. Acute hemorrhagic pancreatitis.

    D. Perforated peptic ulcer.

    E. Ruptured pancreatic pseudocyst.

35. An 18-year-old woman has a 2-cm, firm, rubbery mass in her left breast that moves easily with palpation. The mass is not tender, and she has no other symptoms. This is most likely:

    A. Adenocarcinoma.

    B. Cystosarcoma phyllodes.

    C. Fibroadenoma.

    D. Fibrocystic disease.

    E. Intraductal papilloma.

36. A 74-year-old woman reports that her left breast has been swollen and red for a couple of months. She delayed seeking help because she has no pain or fever. Physical examination shows classical "orange peel" appearance, but no discrete masses can be felt. This is most likely:

    A. Chronic cystic mastitis.

    B. Inflammatory cancer of the breast.

    C. Normal menopausal involutionary changes.

    D. Pyogenic breast abscess.

    E. Tuberculous or fungal breast abscess.

37. A 32-year-old woman in the second month of pregnancy is found to have a 2-cm mass in her left breast. Mammogram shows no other lesions, and core biopsies reveal infiltrating ductal carcinoma. The best course of action would be:

    A. Appropriate surgical excision now, deferring other therapeutic modalities.

    B. Breast surgery, chemotherapy, and radiation at this time.

    C. Chemotherapy now, deferring surgery until after delivery.

    D. Immediate therapeutic abortion and palliative breast surgery.

    E. Radiotherapy now, deferring surgery until after delivery.

38. A 39-year-old woman discovers a lump on her lower neck that goes up and down with swallowing. Physical examination discloses a 2-cm, firm mass in the right lobe of her thyroid gland. She is otherwise asymptomatic. The appropriate course of action for this mass will best be established by:

    A. Careful observation over the next few years.

    B. Fine-needle aspiration (FNA) cytology of the mass.

    C. Radionuclide scan of the thyroid gland.

    D. Response to suppression by exogenous thyroid medication.

    E. Thyroid function tests (T4 and TSH).

39. An asymptomatic 44-year-old woman is persuaded to have her blood pressure checked at a health fair sponsored by her church. She is found to be hypertensive, which surprises her, because "I have always been healthy, and I'm not on any medications." Her physical examination is otherwise unremarkable, but the lab reports slight elevations of serum sodium and bicarbonate, and serum potassium of 2.3 mEq per liter. The next study should be:

    A. Cortisol byproducts in the urine.

    B. Serum aldosterone and renin.

    C. Serum and urinary catecholamines.

    D. Somatomedin C.

    E. Split renal function.

40. Within 8 hours of birth, it is noted that a baby has excessive salivation. A small, soft nasogastric tube is inserted, and the baby is taken to x-ray for a "babygram." The film shows the NG tube coiled back upon itself in the upper chest and air in the gastrointestinal tract. The presumptive diagnosis at this time is:

    A. Complete discontinuity of the esophagus, with no T-E fistula.

    B. Congenital diaphragmatic hernia.

    C. Duodenal atresia.

    D. H-type tracheoesophageal fistula.

    E. Proximal esophageal atresia with distal tracheoesophageal fistula.

41. A 3-day-old, full-term baby boy is brought in because of feeding intolerance and bilious vomiting. X-rays show multiple dilated loops of small bowel and a "ground glass" appearance in the lower abdomen. The child's mother has cystic fibrosis. Which of the following is a diagnostic test that would also have therapeutic value for this infant?

    A. Barium enema.

    B. Colonoscopy.

    C. Endoscopic retrograde cholangiopancreatography (ERCP).

    D. Full thickness rectal biopsy.

    E. Gastrografin enema.

42. The parents of a 6-month-old baby boy report that their son has two problems. At times he has stridor, crowing respiration, and respiratory distress, during which he hyperextends his neck. He also seems to have some difficulty swallowing. Bronchoscopy shows segmental tracheal compression and rules out tracheomalacia. A barium swallow shows extrinsic compression upon the esophagus. Correction of this baby's anomaly will be achieved by:

    A. Endoscopic fulguration of congenital webs.

    B. Surgical division and repositioning of the trachea.

    C. Surgical division of an abnormal blood vessel.

    D. Surgical enlargement of the thoracic inlet.

    E. Surgical rerouting of the esophagus.

43. A 22-year-old man shows up at the ER with obvious congestive heart failure, which he says he developed in just a few days. When his private cardiologist saw him recently for a regular check-up, his heart was normal. He has fever and a loud diastolic murmur at the right second intercostal space, and his blood pressure is 130 over 20. He is a wealthy young man who admits to self-administering intravenous heroin. This man will need:

    A. Closure of ventricular septic defect with a pericardial patch.

    B. Elective aortic valve repair if he develops a 50 mm gradient.

    C. Emergency aortic valve replacement and long-term antibiotics.

    D. Emergency mitral valve repair and long-term antibiotics.

    E. Emergency pulmonic valve commissurotomy.

44. A 73-year-old chronic smoker has a chest x-ray as part of his ongoing medical care for very severe COPD. The film shows a new central hilar mass, and bronchoscopy and biopsies have diagnosed squamous cell carcinoma. He has FEV_1 of 1,100, and 55% of lung function comes from the affected lung, according to a ventilation-perfusion scan. In order to determine operability, this man needs:

    A. CT scan to rule out liver metastasis.

    B. Endobronchial ultrasound to biopsy carinal nodes.

    C. Mediastinal exploration via a collar incision.

    D. No further tests; he is a good candidate for palliative pneumonectomy.

    E. No further tests; he is not a surgical candidate.

45. A 39-year-old male known to have atrial fibrillation has sudden onset of pain in his entire right lower extremity. The leg is cold, pulseless, and paresthetic, and he cannot move it. He arrived at the ER within an hour of the onset of his symptoms. He will need to be treated with:

    A. Dacron prosthetic vascular conduits.

    B. Fogarty catheters.

    C. Heparin and dicumarol.

    D. Saphenous vein bypasses.

    E. Selective sympathetic blocks.

46. A 65-year-old West Texas farmer of Swedish ancestry has an indolent, raised, waxy 1.2-cm skin mass over the bridge of the nose that has been slowly growing over the past 3 years. There are no enlarged lymph nodes in the head and neck. This is a pretty good description for a:

    A. Basal cell carcinoma.

    B. Invasive melanoma.

    C. Pyogenic granuloma.

    D. Squamous cell carcinoma.

    E. Superficial melanoma.

47. Very reliable parents bring in a 4-year-old boy because in the last 6 months he has developed strabismus. Indeed, his eyes both look inward. Treatment for this child should be:

    A. Based on the use of corrective lenses.

    B. Considered only for cosmetic reasons.

    C. Delayed until puberty.

    D. Done as soon as possible to avoid amblyopia.

    E. Done if spontaneous correction has not occurred by age 7.

48. A 15-year-old girl has a round, 1-cm cystic mass in the midline of her neck at the level of the hyoid bone. When the mass is palpated at the same time that the tongue is pulled, there seems to be a connection between the two. The mass has been present for at least 10 years but only recently bothered the patient because it got infected. The most likely diagnosis is:

    A. Branchial cleft cyst.

    B. Cystic hygroma.

    C. Epidermal inclusion cyst.

    D. Metastatic thyroid cancer.

    E. Thyroglossal duct cyst.

49. A 69-year-old man who smokes and drinks and has rotten teeth has a unilateral, right-sided earache that has not gone away in 6 weeks. Physical examination shows serous otitis media on the right side, but not on the left. Palpation inside his mouth shows induration in the area where the right eustachian tube opens into the pharynx. The diagnosis of his problem will most likely be established by:

    A. Audiometry.

    B. Biopsies of the tympanic membrane and ear canal.

    C. Cultures of fluid aspirated from the affected middle ear.

    D. MRI studies of the eighth nerve.

    E. Panendoscopy (triple endoscopy) and biopsies.

50. A fully conscious 55-year-old man is brought to the ER from the scene of an auto accident. Because he has multiple fractures to the face and base of the skull, a resident checks the function of his cranial nerves. The resident's note records that both seventh nerves are functioning normally. By the next morning, the patient has developed unilateral facial nerve paralysis. What is the most likely cause of this new finding, and what should be done about it?

    A. Edema compressing the nerve; no specific therapy.

    B. Leaking cerebrospinal fluid; antibiotics.

    C. Nerve entrapment; surgical decompression.

    D. Nerve transection; surgical repair.

    E. Viral infection; antivirals.

51. A 38-year-old woman is sick and tired of sitting up in bed all night, taking digitalis and diuretics, and being short of breath all the time. She asks if surgery could be done to help her. At age 18 she had rheumatic fever, and for the past 6 years she has suffered from progressive dyspnea on exertion, orthopnea, paroxysmal nocturnal dyspnea, cough, and hemoptysis. She looks thin and cachectic, and she has atrial fibrillation and a low-pitched, rumbling, diastolic apical murmur. The preferred procedure would be:

    A. Closure of the ventricular septal defect.

    B. Mitral annuloplasty to tighten her incompetent mitral valve.

    C. Mitral commissurotomy to open a stenotic mitral valve.

    D. Prosthetic replacement of the aortic valve.

    E. Prosthetic replacement of the mitral valve.

52. Because of an episode of hemoptysis, a chest x-ray is done on a 66-year-old chronic smoker. A previously nonexistent central hilar mass is discovered, and biopsy via bronchoscopy diagnoses squamous cell carcinoma. The patient has an FEV_1 of 1,950, and a ventilation-perfusion scan shows that 40% of pulmonary function comes from the affected lung. Further workup should:

    A. Assess cardiac risk, because pneumonectomy is indicated.

    B. Be directed at establishing the subtype of cancer.

    C. Be directed at evaluating the presence or absence of metastasis.

    D. Not be done, because he cannot tolerate a pneumonectomy.

    E. Not be done, because the proper treatment is not surgical.

53. A 75-year-old hypertensive woman has extremely severe chest pain of sudden onset. She reports pain that feels like tearing, radiates to the back, and migrated down shortly after it began. When seen in the ER she has a blood pressure of 225 over 115, unequal pulses in the upper extremities, and a wide mediastinum on chest x-ray. She has a creatinine of 4, and EKG and cardiac enzymes rule out a myocardial infarction. The next step in her management should be:

    A. Emergency MRI angiogram.

    B. Gastrografin swallow, followed by barium if negative.

    C. Pulmonary angiography.

    D. Spiral CT scan enhanced with intravenous dye (CT angio).

    E. Ventilation-perfusion scan.

54. A 75-year-old farmer of Irish ancestry who has lived all his life in Alice, Texas, has a nonhealing, indolent 4-cm ulcer over the left temple. The ulcer is punched-out and clean-looking and has been slowly growing over the past 3 years. There are no enlarged lymph nodes in the head or neck. Proper management would best be dictated by:

    A. Full thickness biopsy at the center of the lesion.

    B. Full thickness biopsy at the edge of the lesion.

    C. Pathological studies after the entire lesion has been resected, with a 2-cm margin all around.

    D. Response to a trial of radiation therapy.

    E. Scrapings and cultures of the ulcer base.

55. The health care provider at the well-baby clinic observes that a 1-year-old child has a white pupil on the right side. Fearing a possible retinoblastoma, the provider requests an ophthalmological consultation. This report reads, "Leukocoria due to congenital cataract. Please discuss elective removal with the parents." What is the best response to the parents about the timing of such an operation?

    A. It is already too late to avoid amblyopia.

    B. It is entirely at the discretion of the parents.

    C. Surgery should await possible spontaneous involution.

    D. Surgery should be done as soon as possible to avoid amblyopia.

    E. Surgery should not be done until after age 7.

56. A 17-year-old girl has a 3-cm, fluctuant round mass on the side of her neck, just beneath and in front of the sternomastoid muscle, at the level of the superior edge of the thyroid cartilage. She reports that it has been there all her life but has slowly grown to its present size over the past few years. A curious physical finding is a little dimple on the skin, right over the mass. CT scan shows the mass to be cystic. This is probably a:

   A. Branchial cleft cyst.

   B. Cystic hygroma.

   C. Metastatic tumor.

   D. Necrotic lymphoma.

   E. Thyroglossal duct cyst.

57. A 53-year-old man complains of hearing loss. When tested with a tuning fork, he is found to have unilateral sensory hearing loss, affecting the right side only. He is right-handed but does not engage in any activity that would expose that side to loud noise that would not affect the opposite side. He has no other symptoms. Further workup should look for:

   A. A plug of cerumen.

   B. Acoustic nerve neuroma.

   C. Hemorrhagic cerebrovascular disease.

   D. Ischemic cerebrovascular disease.

   E. Occult parotid tumor.

58. A 42-year-old woman that you have been treating for frontal and ethmoid sinusitis calls your office to report that she is running a high fever, and that she woke up this morning with severe pain in the middle of her face, as well as double vision. This lady will need:

   A. An appointment to see an ophthalmologist.

   B. Emergency craniotomy to drain pus from her cavernous sinus.

   C. In-hospital IV antibiotics and drainage of the paranasal sinuses.

   D. Transnasal surgical extraction of clots from the cavernous sinus.

   E. X-rays of her face to make a proper diagnosis.

59. A 73-year-old man suddenly loses vision from his left eye and cannot move the right half of his body. Within minutes, he is taken by ambulance to a local hospital that has been designated as the medical facility staffed and equipped to treat ongoing strokes. The man is conscious but frightened and confused, and he cannot say whether he has a headache or not. The next step in his management should be:

   A. Arteriogram to identify and embolize the source of intracranial bleeding.

   B. CT scan of his head to rule out intracranial bleeding or very extensive infarct.

   C. Intravenous infusion of tissue-type plasminogen activator (t-PA).

   D. Make arrangements to treat with t-PA if he has not recovered after 3 hours.

   E. Spinal tap to rule out subarachnoid bleeding.

60. A 15-year-old girl has gained weight and "become ugly." She brings a picture of herself, taken a year ago, showing a lovely-looking young woman. Now she has a hairy, red, round face full of pimples; her neck has a posterior fat hump; and her supraclavicular areas are round and convex. She has a fat trunk and thin extremities, as well as mild diabetes and hypertension. Which of the following tests will eventually help establish a diagnosis?

    A. Aldosterone and renin determinations.

    B. Dexamethasone suppression tests.

    C. MRI of the adrenal glands.

    D. Urinary collection of catecholamines.

    E. Urinary collection for 5-hydroxyindoleacetic acid.

61. A 60-year-old man complains of extremely severe, sharp shooting pain in his face, "like a bolt of electricity." The pain is brought about by touching a specific area and occurs many times during the day, each episode lasting about 60 seconds. Neurologic exam is normal, but it is noted that part of his face is unshaven because he fears touching that area. Once organic lesions have been ruled out with an MRI, treatment should begin with:

    A. Carbamazepine.

    B. Glucosamine.

    C. Ibuprofen.

    D. Oxycodone.

    E. Steroids.

62. A 23-year-old man presents in the ER with extremely severe testicular pain, of recent onset. He has fever of 103°F and pyuria. The affected testis is in the normal position, appears to be swollen, and is extremely tender to palpation. The cord above the testis is equally tender. Gently supporting and lifting the scrotal contents affords slight relief from the pain. The proper management includes:

A. Antiviral medications.

B. Emergency surgery and bilateral orchiopexy.

C. Sonogram and antibiotics.

D. Trans-scrotal biopsy.

E. Unilateral testicular resection.

63. A 16-year-old boy goes on a beer-drinking binge for the first time in his life and shortly thereafter develops severe, colicky flank pain. This is a classic scenario for:

A. Bladder calculi.

B. Low implantation of one ureter.

C. Ureteropelvic junction obstruction.

D. Urethral stone.

E. Vesicoureteral reflux.

64. A pre-employment chest x-ray shows a large peripheral coin lesion in a 25-year-old man. Physical exam discloses a hard testicular mass, and orchiectomy by the inguinal route provides a diagnosis of seminoma. Further therapy for this young man should include:

    A. Contralateral orchiectomy.

    B. Cyclophosphamide.

    C. 5-FU and methotrexate.

    D. Only palliative care because his prognosis is hopeless.

    E. Platinum-based chemotherapy.

65. A 66-year-old diabetic man with generalized arteriosclerotic occlusive disease reports gradual loss of erectile function. At first he could get erections, but they did not last long; later the quality of the erections was poor; and eventually there were no erections at all. With the use of a short strip of postage stamps from a perforated roll, it is shown that he has no nocturnal erections either. The first line of therapy in this man should be:

    A. Implantable prosthesis.

    B. Nerve reconstruction.

    C. Psychotherapy.

    D. Sildenafil (Viagra).

    E. Vascular surgery.

66. Ten days after a cadaveric liver transplantation and initiation of a standard immunosuppressive regimen, the 55-year-old recipient begins to have elevated levels of gamma glutamyl transferase, alkaline phosphatase, and bilirubin. Workup should start with:

    A. Determination of portal pressures.

    B. Liver biopsy.

    C. Rechecking of ABO matching.

    D. Trial of steroid boluses.

    E. Ultrasound and Doppler studies.

67. A 46-year-old man involved in a severe automobile collision arrives in the ER unconscious with multiple facial fractures, brisk bleeding into his nose and mouth, and gurgly, irregular, and noisy breathing. Several attempts at endotracheal intubation have failed because the blood obscures the view and the nose does not have a lumen anymore. Five minutes have passed. It is time to do:

    A. Cricothyroidotomy.

    B. Emergency percutaneous tracheostomy over a light source.

    C. Emergency tracheostomy via a collar incision at the base of the neck.

    D. High-frequency ventilation by facial mask.

    D. Percutaneous needle insertion into the upper thyroid notch.

68. A young woman has been stabbed in the chest with a 6-inch-long kitchen knife. She has an entry wound just to the left of the sternal border, at the fourth intercostal space. Her blood pressure is 80 over 50, her pulse rate is 110, and she is cold, pale, and perspiring heavily. She has big, distended veins in her face and neck, but she is breathing normally and has bilateral breath sounds. The next step in management should be:

    A. Administer diuretics to lower the venous congestion.

    B. Empty the pericardial sac by the most expeditious means.

    C. Get a chest x-ray to establish a proper diagnosis.

    D. Place bilateral chest tubes.

    E. Suture the laceration on her chest wall.

69. A pedestrian is hit by a car. He arrives in the ER in coma. He has clear fluid dripping from the left ear and a dark bruise behind his ear and over his left mastoid area. As he is being taken to the CT scanner for a scan of the head, you would recommend that:

    A. He first be given high-dose corticosteroids.

    B. He first be placed on antibiotics.

    C. The CT scan be deferred until he is no longer leaking cerebrospinal fluid.

    D. The CT be extended to include his neck.

    E. The CT scan be preceded by cervical spine x-rays.

70. A 19-year-old male is shot once in the neck with a .22-caliber revolver. It is obvious from the location of the entrance wound and the location of the bullet in x-rays that the entire trajectory lies above the level of the angle of the mandible, but the bullet has not entered the skull. The patient is not yet in shock, but his blood pressure has been slowly declining. Further evaluation would best be done by:

    A. Arteriogram.

    B. Barium studies.

    C. Continued clinical observation.

    D. Endoscopy.

    E. Surgical exploration.

71. You are checking a newborn baby boy in the nursery as his father anxiously watches the proceedings. One of the baby's testicles is in the canal, rather than the scrotum. You can easily pull it down to its proper location, but it will not stay there: It snaps right back up. The father has heard about undescended testicles and asks you what should be done with his child. You explain to him that:

    A. If it has not descended by 1 year, the boy will need an orchiopexy.

    B. Hormonal therapy will hasten the testicular descent.

    C. The child should be worked up for chromosomal abnormalities.

    D. We no longer believe that undescended testicles become malignant.

    E. What his child has is a hyperactive cremasteric muscle.

72. A 31-year-old woman crashes her car against a bridge abutment. She has multiple injuries, including upper and lower extremity fractures. Her blood pressure is 135 over 75, and her pulse rate is 82. On physical exam she has a rigid, tender abdomen with guarding and rebound on all quadrants. The next step in management should be:

    A. CT scan of the abdomen.

    B. Continued clinical observation.

    C. Diagnostic peritoneal lavage.

    D. Exploratory laparotomy.

    E. Sonogram of the abdomen.

73. A 22-year-old man is shot twice in the abdomen with a .22-caliber handgun. One entry wound lies to the left of the umbilicus, with the bullet lodged in the right psoas muscle. The second entry wound is just above the pubis, and that bullet is in the middle of his abdomen. He has gross hematuria. Evaluation of the hematuria would best be done by:

    A. CT scan of the abdomen.

    B. Cystoscopy.

    C. Exploratory laparotomy.

    D. Intravenous pyelogram.

    E. Retrograde urethrogram.

74. The mother of a 1-year-old child brings him in because she has felt a mass in the baby's abdomen. While she cradles and pacifies him, you can palpate a mass in the right upper quadrant that clearly moves up and down with respiration. You plan to do imaging studies, but right now you suspect—and you therefore also want to measure:

    A. Benign liver hemangioma; unconjugated bilirubin.

    B. Choledochal cyst; bilirubin and alkaline phosphatase.

    C. Malignant tumor of the liver; alpha fetoprotein.

    D. Neuroblastoma of the right adrenal gland; catecholamine by-products in the urine.

    E. Wilms tumor of the right kidney; red cells in the urine.

75. A 53-year-old woman comes in because of a breast mass. Two days ago she noticed a lump on self-examination. She has a 2-cm, firm, nontender mass in the left breast, which is movable within the breast. She has no prior history of breast disease, but she is a well-read and well-informed patient who gets regular screening mammograms. She is due for her next one in 3 months. The next step in management should be:

    A. Do fine-needle aspiration (FNA), and nothing more if no cancer cells are seen.

    B. Do mammographically or sonographically guided core biopsies.

    C. Do surgical excision of the mass.

    D. Wait one full menstrual cycle for possible spontaneous resolution.

    E. Wait for the mammogram that she is already scheduled for.

76. You get a phone call from a frantic mother. Her 7-year-old girl spilled Liquid-Plumr all over her arms and legs. You can hear the girl screaming in pain in the background. You should instruct the mother to:

    A. Cover the burned areas with triple antibiotic ointment.

    B. Get the girl in the shower and wash her for at least 30 minutes before bringing her in.

    C. Get the girl to the ER as soon as possible.

    D. Wash the burned areas with diluted vinegar.

    E. Wrap the burned areas in sterile dressings before coming to the ER.

77. Three hours ago, a 72-kg man sustained second- and third-degree flame burns to an estimated 35% of his body surface. Ringer lactate without sugar has been infused at a rate of 1 liter per hour, and his urinary output has been measured by an indwelling catheter. In those first 3 hours his urinary output was 290 mL/h, 315 mL/h, and 350 mL/h. Based on that information, you should:

    A. Administer diuretics.

    B. Continue the infusion at the same rate.

    C. Decrease the rate of fluid administration.

    D. Start using dextrose-containing solutions.

    E. Switch from Ringer lactate to plasma.

78. During a wilderness trek at a national park, a young woman inadvertently bumps into a beehive and is repeatedly stung by a swarm of angry bees. She is rushed to the first aid station, where she is found to be wheezing, hypotensive, and madly scratching an urticarial rash. The drug of choice in this setting is:

    A. Alpha-blocker.

    B. Antivenin.

    C. Dopamine.

    D. Epinephrine.

    E. Propanolol.

79. A 5-year-old boy is brought in by concerned parents because he is "knock-kneed." Indeed he is, although he appears to be quite happy and has no complaints. The parents should be:

    A. Advised that corrective shoes will solve the problem.

    B. Asked to consent to appropriate x-ray studies.

    C. Reassured that this is normal.

    D. Told that the child has Blount disease and needs surgery.

    E. Told that the growth plate must be defective.

80. A 68-year-old woman arrives in the ER with a clinically obvious fracture of the radius and a possible dislocation of the ulnar stylus process. When questioned about the trauma that caused the injury, the woman reports that there was none: She attempted to lift a heavy bag of groceries, and "My arm broke." You immediately suspect:

    A. Metastatic osteolytic cancer.

    B. Osteitis fibrosa cystica from parathyroid disease.

    C. Osteomalacia from nutritional deficiency.

    D. Osteoporosis.

    E. Primary malignant bone tumor (osteogenic sarcoma).

81. A 36-year-old man comes in complaining of wrist pain. He says that he fell on his outstretched hand, and on physical exam he is distinctly tender when you press over his anatomic snuff-box. X-rays of the area are read as negative. The diagnosis and appropriate management are:

    A. Carpal navicular (scaphoid) fracture; thumb spica cast.

    B. De Quervain tenosynovitis; steroid injections.

    C. Ligamentous injury; ace bandages and analgesics.

    D. Nothing broken or damaged; reassurance.

    E. Radial bone hairline fracture; no specific therapy needed.

82. A 22-year-old football player has to be carted off the field after his knee is injured. He has severe knee pain and swelling. You sit him at the edge of the examination table with his legs dangling, then grasp and pull the affected leg. It extends toward you as if you were opening a drawer. The injured structure is:

    A. Anterior cruciate ligament.

    B. Lateral collateral ligament.

    C. Medial collateral ligament.

    D. Medial meniscus.

    E. Posterior cruciate ligament.

83. The front-seat passenger in a car crash is brought to the ER. He was not wearing a seatbelt, and he states that he hit the dashboard with his knees and complains of pain in his right hip. He lies in the stretcher in the ER with the right lower extremity shortened, adducted, and internally rotated. He probably has:

    A. A sprain of some sort that is not an emergency.

    B. Femoral neck fracture.

    C. Intertrochanteric fracture.

    D. Posterior dislocation of the hip.

    E. Posterior dislocation of the knee.

84. A 77-year-old man wants to know if something can be done to improve the function of his right hand. The hand is contracted, and palmar fascial nodules are readily palpable. In casual conversation, he mentions that his parents were Norwegian immigrants. The most likely diagnosis is:

    A. Carpal tunnel syndrome.

    B. De Quervain tenosynovitis.

    C. Dupuytren contracture.

    D. Palmar tenosynovitis.

    E. Rheumatoid arthritis.

85. A 67-year-old man has had an indolent, nonhealing ulcer at the heel of the right foot for several weeks. The ulcer base looks dirty, and there is hardly any granulation tissue. The patient began wearing a new pair of shoes shortly before the ulcer started and noticed a blister where the ulcer eventually developed, but he was not concerned because he felt no pain at all in that area. Dorsalis pedis pulses are palpable. He is obese, has high cholesterol, and has poorly controlled type 2 diabetes mellitus. The events leading to the ulcer can be summarized as:

    A. Allergy to leather, inflammatory response, necrosis.

    B. Arteriosclerosis, large vessel disease, ischemic ulceration.

    C. Diabetic neuropathy, pressure point, small vessel disease.

    D. Infection, poor immune response, fungal tissue destruction.

    E. Venous insufficiency, edema, induration, ulceration.

86. A 66-year-old man with advanced cirrhosis of the liver has been bleeding on and off from a duodenal ulcer. He is being evaluated for possible surgical intervention. Clinically, he has ascites and encephalopathy. The lab reports total bilirubin 4.2, INR of 2 (prothrombin time 28), and serum albumin 2.4. Further management should be:

    A. Administration of albumin prior to surgery.

    B. Administration of vitamin K prior to surgery.

    C. Dialysis to lower the bilirubin prior to surgery.

    D. All the three steps outlined above, then surgery.

    E. An alternative therapy, because he is not a surgical candidate.

87. A 57-year-old man has had an exploratory laparotomy for a gunshot wound of the abdomen. He had 2 bullet holes in the small bowel that were easily repaired. The bullet was embedded in the psoas muscle, and no effort was made to remove it. The abdomen was thoroughly irrigated after surgery, and his abdominal closure left the skin open. His urinary bladder had to be catheterized twice post-op because he could not void. He has been walking since day 1, and began oral fluids on day 3. That evening he developed a fever spike to 103°F; he had been afebrile on days 1 and 2. The most likely diagnosis is:

    A. Atelectasis.

    B. Deep thrombophlebitis.

    C. Intraabdominal abscess.

    D. Urinary tract infection.

    E. Wound infection.

88. A 21-year-old male has had multiple problems while in the ICU recovering from a laparotomy for a gunshot wound. Initially, his chest x-rays and respiratory function were normal, but he now has bilateral pulmonary infiltrates and a PO_2 of 65 while breathing 40% oxygen. There is no evidence of congestive heart failure. The diagnosis and appropriate therapy are:

A. Adult respiratory distress syndrome; positive-end expiratory pressure (PEEP).

B. Aspiration pneumonia; bronchoscopy and lavage.

C. Fat embolism; steroids.

D. Pneumonia; antibiotics.

E. Pulmonary failure; long-term 100% oxygen by mask.

89. A 58-year-old man who had presented with pneumaturia had a laparotomy for resection of the sigmoid colon and repair of the urinary bladder. The postoperative diagnosis was colovesical fistula secondary to diverticulitis, and the incision used was a lower midline. On the fifth postoperative day, you are called to see him because he has been soaking his dressings with large amounts of clear salmon-pink-colored fluid with no particular odor. The Foley catheter has been draining normally. At this time you should:

A. Ask him to get up and go to the examining room for a good look at his incision.

B. Culture the fluid and start empiric antibiotic therapy.

C. Remove the dressings and probe the wound until pus is found and drained.

D. Stop all oral feedings and begin parenteral nutrition.

E. Tape and bind the wound securely while planning surgical reclosure.

90. A 71-year-old man comes in with severe diabetic ketoacidosis, profound dehydration, and a serum potassium concentration of 5.2 mEq/L. After several hours of vigorous therapy with insulin and rehydration with normal saline, his serum potassium concentration is reported as 2.9 mEq/L. That marked difference is best explained as due to:

    A. Correction of acidosis and return of potassium to the cells.

    B. Dilution due to volume correction.

    C. Laboratory error.

    D. Renal exchange of sodium for potassium.

    E. Renal failure due to dehydration.

91. A 44-year-old man comes to the ER at 2:00 a.m. because he just vomited a large amount of bright red blood. When you approach him to take a history, he reeks of alcohol. He gives you a remarkably lucid account of drinking at several bars, then having a couple of hours of vomiting and retching that brought up only clear fluid, and finally vomiting the bloody emesis. This is a pretty good description of:

    A. Bleeding esophageal varices.

    B. Erosive gastritis.

    C. Esophageal perforation (Boerhaave syndrome).

    D. Mallory-Weiss tear.

    E. Stress ulceration.

92. A 58-year-old man gives a history of 2 months of increasing constipation and a remarkable change in the appearance of his stools. They are no longer "like cigars" but have become flat, like a ribbon. Most alarmingly, for a few weeks now he has seen bright red blood coating the outside of those flat stools. The most likely diagnosis is:

    A. Anal fissure.

    B. Cancer of the cecum.

    C. Cancer of the rectum.

    D. Condyloma acuminata of the anus.

    E. Internal hemorrhoids.

93. An emaciated 29-year-old, HIV-positive man, who is the receptive member of a homosexual couple, states that for several months he has been having bloody bowel movements. Physical exam yields two impressive findings: He has a fungating mass growing out of his anus, and his inguinal nodes are enlarged and rock hard on both sides. He probably has:

    A. Adenocarcinoma of the rectum.

    B. Condyloma acuminata of the anus.

    C. External hemorrhoids.

    D. Rectal prolapse.

    E. Squamous cell carcinoma of the anus.

94. A 50-year-old woman is lying motionless on a stretcher in the ER. She is obviously in extreme pain, which she says came on suddenly and is generalized all over her belly. She is very reluctant to be touched, but you gently ascertain that she has a rigid abdomen, with muscle guarding and rebound on all quadrants and no bowel sounds. A CT scan taken before you were called shows free air under the diaphragm. The diagnosis is:

A. Acute obstruction of some intraabdominal viscera.

B. An acute abdomen, the nature of which cannot be defined.

C. An acute inflammatory process in the abdomen.

D. Perforation somewhere in the GI tract.

E. Rupture of a fluid collection with chemical peritonitis.

95. A 44-year-old woman is recovering from an episode of acute ascending cholangitis, secondary to choledocholithiasis. She develops fever and leukocytosis with some tenderness in the right upper quadrant. There is minimal elevation of the liver function tests, and a sonogram shows normal-size biliary ducts and a liver abscess 8 cm in diameter. Therapy for this patient will be centered on:

A. ERCP and sphincterotomy.

B. Long-term intravenous antibiotics.

C. Metronidazole.

D. Open surgical resection of the affected lobe.

E. Percutaneous drainage of the liver abscess.

96. An obese 44-year-old white woman comes in with a history of episodes of nausea, vomiting, and colicky right upper quadrant abdominal pain that radiates to the right shoulder and around to the back. She says the pain usually starts after she eats fatty food, and often it goes away spontaneously in less than an hour. If not, one of her older 5 children takes her to an urgent care clinic, where she is given anticholinergics and gets better. This patient is completely asymptomatic right now, and her physical exam is unremarkable. The next step in management should be:

    A. Counseling the patient to avoid greasy foods.

    B. Endoscopy of the upper GI tract.

    C. Magnetic resonance imaging (MRI) of the upper abdomen.

    D. Sonogram of the right upper quadrant.

    E. Upper GI series with barium.

97. A 9-month-old baby girl is brought in because she has an umbilical hernia. The defect is 1 cm in diameter, and the contents are freely reducible. You recommend:

    A. Elective laparoscopic surgical repair.

    B. Elective open surgical repair.

    C. No therapy unless the hernia persists beyond age 2.

    D. Repeated injections of sclerosing agents.

    E. Urgent surgical repair.

98. A 79-year-old woman has a firm, movable 3-cm mass in her left breast, which has been present for 4 months. She was seen elsewhere a month ago, and she brings a report that essentially says her mammogram is not diagnostic of cancer but cannot rule it out either. The next step in management should be:

    A. Excision of the mass in the operating room.

    B. Fine needle aspiration (FNA) of the mass.

    C. Radiographically guided core biopsies.

    D. Reassurance and a follow-up visit scheduled in 1 year.

    E. Repeat the mammogram in 1 month.

99. A 63-year-old woman has a 4-cm mass just under the nipple and areola of her right breast. Her breast is small and the mass occupies most of it, although it can be easily moved from the chest wall. She had multiple core biopsies taken at a breast imaging center, and the diagnosis is infiltrating ductal carcinoma. She has no other lesions, and physical exam of the axilla is negative. The most appropriate surgical component of her treatment is:

    A. Lumpectomy alone.

    B. Lumpectomy and axillary sampling.

    C. Lumpectomy with axillary dissection, removing all nodes.

    D. Mastectomy and sentinel node axillary sampling.

    E. Mastectomy with complete emptying of the axillary nodes.

100. A 33-year-old woman has been having constant pain in her back for the past 3 weeks, and physical exam reveals two well-circumscribed areas in her thoracic spine that are tender to palpation. She had a lumpectomy for breast cancer a year ago, followed by chemotherapy and radiation. She is currently on tamoxifen. The nature of this patient's problem could best be diagnosed with:

    A. AP and lateral chest x-rays.

    B. Magnetic resonance imaging (MRI).

    C. Needle biopsies of the tender areas.

    D. Radionuclide bone scan.

    E. Sonogram of the affected areas.

101. A 44-year-old woman has virulent peptic ulcer disease. Extensive medical management, including the use of proton pump inhibitors and eradication of *H. pylori*, fails to heal her ulcers. She has 3 ulcers in the first and second portions of her duodenum, and she also has watery diarrhea. Given this clinical course, we should:

    A. Biopsy the duodenal ulcers.

    B. Culture the watery stools.

    C. Measure serum gastrin.

    D. Repeat the eradication of *H. pylori* every 2 months.

    E. Replenish her normal gut flora.

102. In the second week of life, a baby girl has protracted vomiting of green fluid. X-rays are done, and the radiologist reports, "Double-bubble sign with normal gas pattern in the rest of the abdomen." This little girl probably has:

    A. Annular pancreas.

    B. Duodenal atresia.

    C. Intestinal atresia.

    D. Malrotation.

    E. Meconium ileus.

103. A 1-year-old baby is referred for treatment of a subdural hematoma. In the admission examination retinal hemorrhages are noted. The most likely diagnosis is:

    A. Fibrinogen deficiency.

    B. Hemophilia.

    C. Platelet functional disorder.

    D. Shaken baby syndrome.

    E. Wallenberg syndrome.

104. A 3-day-old premature baby boy is noted to have a precordial machinery-like murmur. He also has mild pulmonary congestion, a wide pulse pressure, and radiological signs of increased pulmonary blood flow. He is not in congestive failure. This profile makes him a good candidate to be treated with:

    A. Beta blockers.

    B. Decongestants.

    C. Indomethacin.

    D. Radiological closure.

    E. Surgical closure.

105. A 42-year-old woman with systemic breast cancer is determined to be positive for HER-2 receptors. She has not been previously treated. She should be treated with:

    A. Anastrozole.

    B. Chemotherapy alone.

    C. Chemotherapy and trastuzumab (Herceptin).

    D. Tamoxifen.

    E. Trastuzumab (Herceptin) alone.

106. A 68-year-old man is brought to the ER with excruciating back pain that began suddenly 45 minutes ago. He is diaphoretic and has a systolic blood pressure of 90. There is an 8-cm, tender, pulsatile mass deep in his epigastrium, above the umbilicus. Chest x-ray and flat plate of the abdomen are unremarkable. Two years ago he was diagnosed with prostatic cancer and treated with orchiectomy and radiation. At this point the clinical assumption is that he has:

A. Dissecting thoracic aortic aneurysm.

B. Fracture of lumbar pedicles with cord compression.

C. Herniated disc.

D. Metastatic tumor to the lumbar spine.

E. Rupturing abdominal aortic aneurysm.

107. A 32-year-old man has puzzling physical findings suggestive of heart disease. An echocardiogram is done, and the report says that a 5-cm solid tumor is growing out of the wall of the left ventricle. Except for surgical removal of a pigmented skin lesion from the middle of his back 3 years ago, the patient has been in excellent health all his life. He denies rheumatic fever or intravenous drug use. The most likely diagnosis is:

A. Desmoplastic reaction in old endocarditis.

B. Metastatic melanoma.

C. Myxoma.

D. Rhabdomyosarcoma.

E. Vegetation from unrecognized rheumatic disease.

108. A 57-year-old myopic man calls his ophthalmologist's office. For the past 5 days he has been seeing flashes of light at night, when his eyes are closed. Three days ago, he began to see floaters during the day—at first just 2 or 3, but more than 20 now. Finally, when he woke up this morning, there was a dark cloud at the top of his visual field. All of these symptoms are affecting his right eye only, and he reports no pain in or near that eye. He probably has:

   A. Acute angle-closure glaucoma.

   B. Age-related macular degeneration.

   C. Embolic central retinal artery occlusion.

   D. Retinal detachment.

   E. Retinoblastoma.

109. A 72-year-old man presents with a lump in his neck, which he noticed about 4 months ago and has been slowly growing since. The mass is lateral to his upper thyroid notch, and it is now 4 cm in diameter, fixed, and nontender. Examination of his mouth reveals a few stumps of rotten teeth. When questioned on tobacco and alcohol use, the man says that he smokes 2 packs a day and drinks at least a pint of hard liquor daily. The next diagnostic step should be:

   A. Open excisional biopsy of the mass.

   B. Open incisional biopsy of the mass.

   C. Panendoscopy (triple endoscopy) and mucosal biopsies.

   D. Radionuclide scan of the thyroid gland.

   E. Sputum cytology and CT scan of the lungs.

110. The mother of a 2-year-old boy brings him in because "pus is running out of his nose." Although the child resists examination, as he sits on his mother's lap you notice that the foul-smelling fluid is coming out of only one nostril. The mother confirms that the nasal discharge has been happening for about a week. Given the child's age and clinical presentation, you already suspect:

    A. Immunodeficiency.

    B. Juvenile nasopharyngeal angiofibroma.

    C. Maxillary sinusitis.

    D. Nasal foreign body.

    E. Septal perforation.

111. A 57-year-old man seeks help for "dizziness." He says that the problem is triggered by sudden movements of his head, and he then feels that the room is spinning, "like being inside a washing machine." There is no headache or any other neurological deficit. The terrifying episodes gradually go away if he stays very still and does not move his head. The location of his pathology is probably in:

    A. The carotid bifurcation.

    B. The cerebellar cortex.

    C. The cerebral cortex.

    D. The inner ear.

    E. The vertebral arteries.

112. A 42-year-old, right-handed man has a history of progressive speech difficulties and right hemiparesis for 5 months. He has had progressively severe headaches for the last 2 months, which are worse in the mornings. At the time of admission he is confused and vomiting and has blurred vision, papilledema, and diplopia. Shortly thereafter, his blood pressure goes up to 190 over 110 and he develops bradycardia. The rise in his blood pressure is due to:

    A. A brain tumor pressing on the hypothalamus.

    B. A compensatory response to preserve brain perfusion (Cushing reflex).

    C. Deviation of the brain stem.

    D. Release of endorphins.

    E. Shifting of cerebrospinal fluid.

113. A 23-year-old man comes in with otitis media and mastoiditis and is placed on appropriate antibiotics. When he returns in 2 weeks he complains of severe headache, seizures, blurred vision, and projectile vomiting. He says he has had a fever for the past week. The next diagnostic study should be:

    A. CT scan of the head.

    B. Culture of aspirate from the recently affected ear.

    C. Culture of cerebrospinal fluid obtained by spinal tap.

    D. Radionuclide scans of the mastoid.

    E. X-rays of the paranasal sinuses.

114. A newborn baby boy has not urinated at all during the first 18 hours of life. Physical exam shows a normal meatus and a distended urinary bladder. The child probably has:

    A. Anterior urethral valves.

    B. Low implantation of the ureters.

    C. Normal variant—newborns often do not urinate until day 2 or 3.

    D. Posterior urethral valves.

    E. Renal agenesis.

115. On a routine physical exam, a 65-year-old man is found to have a 1.5-cm, rock-hard mass in his prostate. His PSA is normal for his age. The next step in management is to:

    A. Do a transrectal needle biopsy of the mass.

    B. Do a transrectal sonogram of the prostate.

    C. Do a transurethral resection of the prostate (TURP).

    D. Follow the evolution of the mass over the ensuing year.

    E. Repeat his PSA before anything else is done.

116. The CT of a 59-year-old woman with severe ureteral colic shows a 7-mm ureteral stone at the ureteropelvic junction. She has a normal coagulation profile. Most urologists would treat this patient with:

    A. Analgesics and plenty of fluids in anticipation of spontaneous passage.

    B. Endoscopic retrograde basket extraction.

    C. Endoscopic retrograde laser vaporization of the stone.

    D. Extracorporeal shock wave lithotripsy.

    E. Open surgical removal.

117. A 4-year-old child has significant blood loss from a gun-shot wound to the left arm. Direct pressure has stanched the bleeding, but fluid resuscitation is urgently needed. Repeated attempts to insert IV lines have been unsuccessful. The best alternate route is:

    A. Central line via subclavian puncture.

    B. Infusion into intracranial sinuses via open fontanelles.

    C. Intraosseous cannulation of the proximal tibia.

    D. Percutaneous femoral vein cannulation.

    E. Saphenous vein cut-down.

118. A spinal anesthetic is placed in a 52-year-old man in preparation for a hemorrhoidectomy. The patient's level of sensory block turns out to be much higher than intended, and he goes into shock. Blood pressure is recorded as 75 over 20, and CVP is near zero. The patient looks warm and flushed. He should be treated with:

   A. Diuretics and fluid restriction.

   B. Inotropic agents and cardiac assist pump.

   C. Vasoconstrictors and intravenous fluids.

   D. Vasodilators and packed red cells.

   E. Whole blood and clotting agents.

119. A 77-year-old man becomes "senile" over a period of 3 or 4 weeks. He used to be active and made an excellent living writing fiction and movie scripts. Now he stares at the wall all day long, barely recognizes his family, and is "a completely different person." Two weeks before the mental changes began, he fell from a horse but apparently sustained no serious injuries. You expect a CT scan of his head to show:

   A. Acute epidural hematoma.

   B. Chronic subdural hematoma.

   C. Diffuse intracranial bleeding.

   D. Frontal lobe infarction.

   E. Generalized brain atrophy.

120. An elderly man is rear-ended in an automobile collision and violently hyperextends his neck. He develops paralysis and burning pain in both upper extremities while maintaining good motor function in his legs. The most likely diagnosis is:

    A. Anterior cord syndrome.

    B. Central cord syndrome.

    C. Posterior cord syndrome.

    D. Reflex sympathetic dystrophy.

    E. Spinal cord hemisection.

121. A 25-year-old man is stabbed in the right chest. He comes in fully awake and alert, and in a normal tone of voice he states that he feels short of breath. His vital signs are normal and stable. On physical exam he has no breath sounds at the right base, and only faint breath sounds at the apex. A chest x-ray confirms that he has a hemothorax on that side. The next step in management should be:

    A. Exploratory thoracotomy.

    B. Insertion of a chest tube aimed at the right base.

    C. Insertion of a 16-gauge needle at the right second intercostal space.

    D. Intubation and use of a respirator.

    E. Oxygen by mask, analgesics, and no specific intervention.

122. The unrestrained front-seat passenger of a car that crashes at high speed arrives at the ER with signs of moderate respiratory distress. Physical exam shows no breath sounds at all on the left hemithorax. Vital signs are normal. Chest x-ray shows a collapsed left lung and multiple air fluid levels filling the left pleural cavity. A nasogastric tube that had been placed prior to taking the film shows the tube reaching the upper abdomen and then curling up into the left chest. Your diagnosis is:

    A. Blowout of pulmonary blebs.

    B. Esophageal rupture or perforation.

    C. Left diaphragmatic rupture.

    D. Left hemopneumothorax.

    E. Major injury to the tracheobronchial tree.

123. A 22-year-old convenience store clerk is shot with a .38-caliber revolver. The entry wound is in the left midclavicular line, 2 inches below the nipple. He is hemodynamically stable, complaining of generalized abdominal pain. Chest x-ray shows a small pneumothorax on the left, free air under both diaphragms, and the bullet lodged in the left paraspinal muscles. In addition to placing a chest tube on the left pleural space, he should also have:

    A. Barium swallow.

    B. Bronchoscopy.

    C. Exploratory laparotomy.

    D. Extraction of the bullet via left thoracotomy.

    E. Extraction of the bullet via local back exploration.

124. A 23-year-old man who sustained multiple injuries in an automobile accident is in shock upon admission. Although he is quickly resuscitated with intravenous fluids, his abdomen is tender all around and rapidly becoming distended. A focused abdominal sonogram for trauma (FAST test) confirms that his abdomen is full of blood. An exploratory laparotomy is quickly started, but he has so many injuries that surgery cannot be finished quickly. By the time everything has been repaired, he has received 12 liters of Ringer lactate and 6 units of packed red cells. When closure of his abdomen is attempted, the swollen edges will not easily come together. The surgeons should:

A. Approximate the skin only, using towel clips.

B. Close the abdomen with heavy retention sutures.

C. Give diuretics and close the abdomen in the usual way.

D. Leave the abdomen and its contents open to the air.

E. Provide temporary bowel coverage with an absorbable mesh.

125. A 22-year-old woman loses control of an all-terrain vehicle (ATV), falls to the ground, and then is crushed when the ATV falls on top of her. She arrives to the ER with stable vital signs but obvious physical evidence of a pelvic fracture. When a Foley catheter is inserted, it recovers bloody urine. The best way to evaluate her urological injury would be:

A. Cystoscopy.

B. Intravenous pyelogram.

C. Retrograde cystogram including post-void films.

D. Retrograde cystogram including views of the ureters.

E. Sonogram of the bladder.

126. A 33-year-old man is shot point-blank in his upper thigh with a .38-caliber revolver. The entrance wound is on the anterio-medial side, and x-rays show the bullet lodged in the muscles, 4 cm farther down. He has a large, expanding hematoma under the entry wound and no pulses below the injury. The next step in management should be:

    A. Arteriogram.

    B. CT angio.

    C. Doppler studies.

    D. Embolectomy with Fogarty catheters.

    E. Surgical exploration and repair.

127. A 57-year-old man weighing 60 kg sustains third-degree burns on both lower extremities. The injury occurred when his pants were accidentally doused with gasoline and ignited, and it appears that no part of either lower extremity was spared. It is decided to begin his fluid resuscitation with a predeter-mined infusion of Ringer lactate without sugar and to adjust the rate of infusion once data about hourly urinary output are obtained. What are the appropriate infusion rate and target urinary output for this patient?

    A. 250 mL/h, aiming for urinary output of 10–40 mL/h.

    B. 500 mL/h, aiming for urinary output of 15–60 mL/h.

    C. 750 mL/h, aiming for urinary output of 25–100 mL/h.

    D. 1,000 mL/h, aiming for urinary output of 30–120 mL/h.

    E. 1,500 mL/h, aiming for urinary output of 45–180 mL/h.

128. During a hunting trip, a young man is bitten on his lower leg by a coyote. The bite drew blood, but the flow was easily stopped by local pressure. The animal was captured and brought alive to the authorities. The need for rabies prophylaxis in this patient should be determined by:

    A. Confining the animal to a cage and watching its behavior.

    B. Cultures of the bite wounds.

    C. Killing the animal and examining the brain.

    D. The patient's clinical course over the next few weeks.

    E. The patient's history of previous childhood immunizations.

129. An obese 13-year-old boy has been limping and complaining of persistent left knee pain for several weeks. He gives no history of trauma. On physical exam his knee is not swollen, and it appears to be entirely normal. However, he has limited hip motion. He sits on the examination table with the sole of his left foot pointing to the right, and when his left hip is passively flexed it goes into external rotation and cannot be rotated internally. The most likely diagnosis is:

    A. Avascular necrosis of the femoral head.

    B. Developmental dysplasia of the hip.

    C. Osteogenic sarcoma of the lower femur.

    D. Slipped capital femoral epiphysis.

    E. Tibial torsion with foot inversion.

130. A 9-year-old girl injures her right forearm. X-rays show that the growth plate is laterally displaced from the metaphysis, but it is not broken. Gentle manipulation easily returns it to its normal location, and a cast is subsequently applied. The likely outcome of such closed reduction in this case is:

    A. Acceptable outcome with no future deformity.

    B. Nerve injury leading to muscle atrophy.

    C. Uneven growth deviating the wrist laterally.

    D. Uneven growth deviating the wrist medially.

    E. Vascular injury leading to Volkmann contracture.

131. A 42-year-old woman comes in with her left arm supported by an improvised sling and held close to her body. She states that when she woke up from an epileptic seizure 2 days ago, she had pain in that shoulder and could not move that arm. She went to an urgent care clinic, where she had AP and lateral x-rays taken and was told they were normal. You suspect—and intend to do:

    A. Anterior dislocation of the shoulder; oblique films.

    B. Acromioclavicular separation; good physical exam.

    C. Articular cartilage crushing; MRI of the shoulder.

    D. Posterior dislocation of the shoulder; axillary or scapular lateral views.

    E. Torn teres major and minor; MRI of the shoulder.

132. A 44-year-old man is brought in from the scene of an automobile accident. He has obvious clinical evidence of bilateral femur fractures, which x-rays show to be comminuted. Shortly after these films are taken, his blood pressure drops to 75 over 55, pulse rate reaches 105, and venous pressure is zero. He has no other pertinent findings. The reason for his hemodynamic situation is:

   A. Blood loss at the fracture sites.

   B. Fat embolism.

   C. Neurogenic shock from pain.

   D. Unrecognized intracranial bleeding.

   E. Unrecognized pericardial tamponade.

133. A 71-year-old man comes in with severe pain and swelling of his right ankle. He states that he lost his footing while going down a steep ladder and landed on his inverted foot. AP, lateral, and mortise x-rays show displaced fractures of both malleoli. He should be treated with:

   A. Closed reduction after the swelling goes down.

   B. Closed reduction and casting now.

   C. Open reduction and internal fixation.

   D. Posterior splint and early ambulation.

   E. Skeletal traction.

134. A 44-year-old man sustains a closed head injury in an automobile accident in which he flew through the windshield and landed on the hood of the car. He is in coma. His pupils are of equal size, and both react to light. He also has scalp lacerations and minor facial scratches. In addition to CT scan of the head, the proper radiological evaluation of this patient should include:

    A. Base of the skull x-rays.

    B. Extension of the CT to include the neck.

    C. MRI of the brain.

    D. Skull x-rays looking for depressed fractures.

    E. X-rays of the maxillary sinuses.

135. A 45-year-old woman attempts the lift a heavy object and suddenly has very severe back and posterior left leg pain, which she describes as "a bolt of electricity." The pain is aggravated by coughing or straining, and it becomes excruciating if her leg is raised while extended. Bladder function, rectal sphincter tone, and perineal sensation are normal. The diagnostic and therapeutic plans should be:

    A. CT scan of entire spine; body cast for 3 months.

    B. Lumbar spine x-rays; strict bed rest for 3 weeks.

    C. MRI centered on L4 to S1; pain control with nerve blocks.

    D. MRI of the lumbar spine; emergency surgical decompression of the cauda equina.

    E. Spinal tap; surgical removal of extruded disc fragments.

136. A 39-year-old West Texas man, who always wears pointed cowboy boots, wants to know if something can be done about a very tender spot that he has between the third and fourth toes. This is most likely:

    A. Bony spur arising from the metatarsal head.

    B. Extraarticular gout.

    C. Ischemic neuropathy.

    D. Morton neuroma.

    E. Plantar fasciitis.

137. A 73-year-old man has a 5.5-cm abdominal aortic aneurysm, for which elective repair has been recommended. In the preoperative evaluation it is noted that he has jugular venous distention. Before he has his operation, he should:

    A. Be evaluated as a candidate for coronary revascularization.

    B. Be given beta-adrenergics and intravenous fluids.

    C. Be placed on anticoagulants.

    D. Have a CT angio of his thoracic aorta.

    E. Receive medical treatment for congestive heart failure.

138. A 38-year-old woman is being prepared for laparoscopic gall-bladder removal under general anesthesia. When she inhales halothane and is injected with succinylcholine, however, her temperature rises to 105°F and the procedure is canceled. Cooling blankets and 100% oxygen are promptly used and emergency lab studies taken, which show metabolic acidosis and hypercalcemia. When the situation is explained to the patient's family, they recall that her grandfather died while having an operation under general anesthesia, but they were never told why that had occurred. She now needs what specific therapy, and monitoring for development of what possible condition?

    A. Bronchodilators; adult respiratory distress syndrome.

    B. Calcium channel blockers; congestive heart failure.

    C. Dantrolene; myoglobinuria.

    D. Fresh frozen plasma; consumption coagulopathy.

    E. Steroids; raised intracranial pressure.

139. On the seventh postoperative day after internal fixation of an intertrochanteric fracture, a 76-year-old man suddenly develops severe pleuritic chest pain and shortness of breath. When examined, he is found to be anxious, diaphoretic, and tachycardic. He has prominent distended veins in his neck and forehead. Blood gases show hypoxemia and hypocapnia. The next steps in management should be:

    A. Aortogram and emergency surgical repair.

    B. EKG, troponins, and clot busters.

    C. Intubation and respirator with hyperventilation and PEEP.

    D. Retinal examination looking for fat droplets.

    E. Spiral CT (CT angio) and heparinization.

140. A 72-year-old man weighing 68 kg had an abdominoperineal resection for cancer of the rectum. An indwelling Foley catheter was left in place after surgery. Although his vital signs have been stable, the nurses are concerned because his Foley catheter output for the last 2 hours has been zero. In the preceding 3 hours they had collected 56 mL, 73 mL, and 67 mL. The most likely diagnosis is:

   A. Acute renal failure.

   B. Damage to the bladder during the operation.

   C. Damage to the ureters during the operation.

   D. Dehydration.

   E. The catheter is plugged or kinked.

141. A group of Mexican nationals are smuggled into the United States in a closed metal truck in the middle of summer. When the U.S. Border Patrol gives chase, the smugglers abandon their charges in the locked truck, in the middle of the desert, with no water to drink. The group is found and rescued 5 days later. One of the victims is delivered to your hospital, awake and alert, with obvious physical findings of severe dehydration and a serum sodium concentration of 155 mEq/L. It is decided to rely on intravenous fluids to correct his problem. Which of the following is the best option?

   A. A total of 3 L normal saline infused over 12 hours.

   B. A total of 4 L 3% saline infused over 8 hours.

   C. A total of 5 L dextrose 5% in half-normal saline infused over 6 hours.

   D. A total of 6 L dextrose 10% in water infused over 4 hours.

   E. A total of 7 L dextrose 5% in water infused over 3 hours.

142. Upper GI endoscopy shows severe peptic esophagitis, Barrett esophagus, and very minimal, early dysplastic changes in a 67-year-old woman with a long history of gastroesophageal reflux disease. This is her fourth endoscopy over the past 10 years. Her best efforts to follow the medical management prescribed by a very competent gastroenterologist have failed. What should we offer her now?

    A. Heller myotomy of the lower esophageal sphincter.

    B. Laparoscopic Nissen fundoplication.

    C. Transhiatal total esophagectomy.

    D. Transthoracic resection of the lower esophagus.

    E. Vagotomy and antrectomy.

143. A 59-year-old man has had protracted vomiting and colicky abdominal pain for 3 days. His abdomen is moderately distended, and he has high-pitched, hyperactive bowel sounds. There is a 5-cm, tender, discolored mass in his left groin. He says that for many years he has had a bulge there that is noticeable when he is walking around and gets bigger when he coughs or strains; it would disappear whenever he was lying down and "pushed it in." But now he cannot push in this mass, and it has been out since he began vomiting. He has fever and leukocytosis. Management at this time requires:

    A. A precise diagnosis made by sonogram of the mass.

    B. A trial of nasogastric suction and IV fluids for a few days.

    C. Insertion of a long rectal tube via sigmoidoscope.

    D. Manual reduction of the hernia and a period of observation.

    E. Urgent surgical intervention.

144. A 23-year-old woman describes exquisite pain with defecation and blood streaks on the outside of the stools. Because of the pain, she avoids having bowel movements and develops constipation, which complicates her problem. She initially refuses physical examination for fear of precipitating the pain. You have an idea of what her problem might be, and thus a reasonable plan of management would be:

   A. Anoscopy regardless of the pain, and quick rubber ligation of hemorrhoids.

   B. Examination under anesthesia, followed by incision and drainage.

   C. Examination under anesthesia, followed by diltiazem ointment.

   D. A follow-up consultation when the patient is feeling better.

   E. Strong laxatives prescribed on the basis of history alone.

145. A 7-year-old boy passed a large bloody bowel movement 2 days ago. He has not bled again since then. Physical examination is noncontributory, and he has a normal hemoglobin level. The diagnostic modality most appropriate to diagnose the source of the bleeding would be:

   A. Arteriogram.

   B. Colonoscopy.

   C. Radioactively labeled technetium scan.

   D. Radioactively tagged red cell study.

   E. Upper GI endoscopy.

146. A 79-year-old man with atrial fibrillation develops an acute abdomen. When seen 3 days after the onset of the abdominal pain, he has a silent abdomen with diffuse tenderness and mild rebound. There is a trace of blood in the rectal exam. He looks quite sick, with acidosis and signs of sepsis. The most likely diagnosis is:

    A. Acute pancreatitis.

    B. Mesenteric ischemia.

    C. Midgut volvulus.

    D. Perforated viscus.

    E. Primary bacterial peritonitis.

147. A 58-year-old woman first noticed scleral icterus 5 weeks ago. Jaundice has been steadily progressing, and now her entire body looks yellow and she has mild itching all over. She also reports vague, constant upper abdominal and back pain and a 10-pound weight loss. The lab reports a total bilirubin of 29, most of which is conjugated (direct) bilirubin. Transaminases are minimally elevated, and alkaline phosphatase is about 5 times the upper limit of normal. An ultrasound of her right upper abdomen shows a thin-walled, massively dilated gallbladder without stones. The next diagnostic procedure should be:

    A. CT scan of the upper abdomen.

    B. Endoscopic retrograde cholangiopancreatogram (ERCP).

    C. Magnetic resonance cholangiopancreatogram (MRCP).

    D. Percutaneous transhepatic cholangiogram.

    E. Sonographically guided endoscopic biopsies.

148. Two weeks after his discharge from the hospital, a 59-year-old, alcoholic man returns, reporting fever and chills for the last 3 days. He was last hospitalized for acute hemorrhagic pancreatitis, and while in the ICU he had pleural effusions and respiratory failure, but he recovered from all of those problems. The only additional finding now is leukocytosis. He has probably developed:

    A. Chronic pancreatitis.

    B. Pancreatic abscess.

    C. Pancreatic pseudocyst.

    D. Pelvic abscess.

    E. Subphrenic abscess.

149. A 27-year-old immigrant from El Salvador has a 14- by 12- by 9-cm mass in her left breast. It has been present for 7 years and has slowly grown to its present size. The mass is firm, rubbery, and completely movable, and it is not attached to overlying skin or the chest wall. There are no palpable axillary nodes. The most likely diagnosis is:

    A. Breast cancer.

    B. Chronic cystic mastitis.

    C. Cystosarcoma phyllodes.

    D. Intraductal papilloma.

    E. Mammary dysplasia.

150. A 54-year-old woman seeks help because she noticed a mass in her left breast. She was actually not in the habit of doing breast self-exams, but she was accidentally hit with a tennis racket, and that brought her attention to the area. She has a 3.5-cm, hard, deep, freely movable mass and some superficial bruising. The next step in management should be:

    A. Fine needle aspiration (FNA).

    B. Mammogram.

    C. Radiologically guided core biopsies.

    D. Reassurance that the trauma is responsible for the mass.

    E. Surgical evacuation of the hematoma.

151. A young man who crashed his Ferrari 2 weeks ago is dying in the intensive care unit with adult respiratory distress syndrome (ARDS) that has failed to respond to conventional therapy. His very wealthy parents are anxious to try whatever new "miracle" procedure might offer hope of survival. He might be a good candidate for:

    A. Extracorporeal membrane oxygenation (ECMO).

    B. Hyperbaric chamber dives at 3 atmospheres of pressure.

    C. Porcine lung graft, as a bridge to bilateral lung allografts.

    D. Repeated infusions of free hemoglobin.

    E. Repeated treatments with standard heart-lung bypass machines.

152. When a premature baby is first fed, he develops signs of feeding intolerance, with abdominal distention and a rapidly dropping platelet count. All feedings are stopped, and the baby is placed on broad-spectrum antibiotics, IV fluids, and IV nutrition. The next day he develops abdominal wall erythema and air in the portal vein. Therapy should now include:

    A. Cannulation of the portal vein for decompression.
    B. Debridement of the abdominal wall.
    C. Intravenous nutrients specifically designed for liver failure.
    D. Parenteral nutrients delivered into the portal vein.
    E. Surgical intervention.

153. A 22-year-old woman comes to the ER with an extremely severe headache that she insists is different from any headache she has ever had before. On direct questioning, she explains that it had sudden onset, denies any history of trauma, and offers no potential explanation for her problem. She still has the headache as she is being examined, but her neurological examination is entirely normal. The next step in management should be:

    A. CT scan of the head.
    B. Psychiatric consultation.
    C. Reassurance and analgesics.
    D. Skull x-rays.
    E. Spinal tap.

154. A 24-year-old woman is surprised to find that she is secreting milk from both breasts, even though she knows perfectly well that she is not pregnant. She suspects some kind of gynecological or endocrine problem, because her menses have been very irregular and now she has amenorrhea. Her workup finds normal TSH, negative pregnancy test, elevated prolactin levels, and the presence of a small pituitary tumor shown on MRI. She is absolutely terrified of the idea of any kind of surgery on her head. She could be offered:

   A. Bromocriptine or a similar drug.

   B. Indomethacin or a similar drug.

   C. Psychiatric counseling, because surgery is her only option.

   D. Radiation therapy.

   E. Watchful waiting, expecting spontaneous involution.

155. A man has been referred to a multidisciplinary clinic because of depression. He explains that he has reason for the way he feels: He was recently fired from his job because of inappropriate behavior; he has been having headaches every morning, and they are getting worse; and lately he has been vomiting for no reason. "I just open my mouth, and the stuff hits the wall," he says. He hardly sees out of one eye, and all foods "taste the same." On neurologic exam he is found to have papilledema on one side, atrophy of the optic nerve on the other, and anosmia. He probably has:

   A. Brain tumor at the base of the frontal lobe.

   B. Brain tumor over the parietal lobe.

   C. Multiple sclerosis.

   D. Senile dementia.

   E. Severe psychiatric problems.

156. A 58-year-old homeless man has been having intermittent hematuria for a year and a half but has not looked for help because "they treat me like trash at the emergency room." Finally he is forced to go when he develops flank pain. Workup shows a flank mass, hypercalcemia, erythrocytosis, and elevated liver enzymes. CT scan shows a heterogenic tumor that has grown into the lumen of the vena cava. This is the full-blown picture of:

    A. Hepatoblastoma.

    B. Prostatic cancer.

    C. Renal cell carcinoma.

    D. Retroperitoneal sarcoma.

    E. Transitional cell carcinoma.

157. A 33-year-old man carelessly removes the radiator cap of his car to find out why the motor is overheating. His face is severely burned with very hot coolant fluid and steam, but fortunately he avoids inhaling the latter. His eyes escaped injury, but he has burns that are very close to them. After everything is cleaned in the operating room, those burns near the eyes should be covered with:

    A. Mafenide acetate.

    B. Petroleum jelly.

    C. Silver sulfadiazine.

    D. Triple antibiotic ointment.

    E. Wet-to-dry dressings.

158. A middle-aged man is brought into the ER with extremely severe abdominal pain of sudden onset. He is thrashing around, trying to get off the stretcher, while his wife attempts to restrain him. This patient probably has:

    A. An inflammatory process in the abdomen.

    B. An ischemic process affecting his bowel.

    C. A perforated hollow viscus.

    D. A stone impacted in his ureter.

    E. Primary bacterial peritonitis.

159. In the course of a mugging, a 27-year-old man is repeatedly kicked in the abdomen. When he is examined in the ER shortly thereafter, he has a blood pressure of 85 over 55 and a pulse rate of 110, with a central venous pressure of 1. Two liters of Ringer lactate are infused over 20 minutes via two 16-gauge catheters, one in each arm. His blood pressure promptly responds, and by the time packed red cells arrive from the blood bank, he is hemodynamically stable. He has no signs of peritoneal irritation on physical exam. The next step in management should be:

    A. CT scan of the abdomen.

    B. Diagnostic peritoneal lavage.

    C. Exploratory laparotomy.

    D. Focused abdominal sonogram for trauma (FAST).

    E. Serial x-rays of the abdomen.

160. A scrawny, pitifully small child is brought in with scalding, mostly second-degree burns of both buttocks. The stepfather indicates that the boy is 3 years old, although he looks no bigger than one and a half. He tells the staff that the child accidentally pulled a pot of boiling water over himself while playing in the kitchen. The most important element in the management of this case will be:

   A. Careful calculation of the fluid needs for the next 24 hours.

   B. Consultation with a nutritionist to improve the child's diet.

   C. Implementation of early excision and grafting.

   D. Referral to the proper authorities for child abuse.

   E. The choice of topical agents to apply to the burned areas.

161. Ten days after a patient receives a cadaveric renal transplant, the new kidney's function begins to deteriorate. A percutaneous biopsy report of the graft reads, "Signs of acute rejection." Management should be:

   A. Antilymphocytic medication (OKT3).

   B. Antithymocyte serum and steroid bolus.

   C. Doppler studies of renal artery and vein.

   D. Gradually increased doses of the baseline immunosuppressants.

   E. Verification that the patient is taking medicines on time.

162. A 72-year-old man has been having irritative voiding symptoms and occasional episodes of hematuria. He worked for many years at a chemical plant, where he suspects he was exposed to carcinogens, and he has seen TV ads from lawyers who promise him a financial bonanza if he sues his former employer. However, except for the fact that he has been smoking 3 packs a day since he was a teenager, an extensive investigation of his occupational environment and his personal habits comes up negative. Repeated urinary cultures and a CT scan of his abdomen have been noncontributory. The next step in management should be:

    A. A trial of therapy with ciprofloxacin.

    B. Cystoscopy.

    C. Intravenous pyelogram.

    D. Intravesical BCG.

    E. Renal biopsies.

163. A 59-year-old man has a ureteral stone impacted just above the point where the ureter empties into the bladder. CT scan shows the stone to measure 3 mm. Although he is having colicky pain, it is relatively mild and he is not nauseous or vomiting. A decision is made to give him plenty of fluids and pain medication, and let him pass the stone. At 3:00 a.m., his doctor gets a call informing him that the patient has developed chills, a fever spike to 105°F, and flank pain. The doctor orders IV antibiotics over the phone. What else should he do?

    A. See the patient in the morning and reevaluate the situation.

    B. Arrange for extracorporeal shock wave lithotripsy to be done tomorrow.

    C. Go to the hospital right now and place a suprapubic tube in the bladder.

    D. Go to the hospital right now and place a nephrostomy tube.

    E. Notify his team that they need to extract that stone by open surgery tomorrow.

164. A 66-year-old obese woman comes in because of a chronic ulcer that she says "does not hurt, but it does not heal either." She has been applying antibiotic creams to no avail. Physical examination shows a 3.5-cm ulcer just above a medial malleolus, with a granulating bed, surrounded by chronically edematous, indurated, hyperpigmented skin. Her obesity precludes any reliable physical examination of her leg veins or her peripheral pulses. An initial plan of treatment should be based on:

    A. Application of ice, bed rest, and elevation.

    B. Biopsy of the ulcer edge followed by resection and radiation treatment.

    C. Doppler studies looking for arterial pressure gradient, and angioplasty or bypass.

    D. Duplex scan of the patient's veins and use of support stockings measured to fit her.

    E. Measurement of HbA1c and strict control of diabetes.

165. A 17-year-old boy has been having right lower quadrant abdominal pain for 2 days. He says the pain began at that location and has been gradually getting worse. On physical exam he has tenderness to deep palpation and mild rebound on both the right lower quadrant and the left lower quadrant. His temperature is 38°C, and his WBC is 8,500. He adds that he is terribly hungry, but his family is afraid to feed him. The next step in management should be:

    A. Barium enema.

    B. CT scan of the abdomen.

    C. Emergency appendectomy.

    D. Lower GI endoscopy.

    E. Trial of antibiotic therapy.

166. A 23-year-old woman has a tubal ligation done under general anesthesia by a vaginal approach. Something goes wrong in the postoperative period, and within a few hours she is in coma. Her records of medications and fluid administrations have been lost, and all we know for sure is that at the time of anesthetic induction her serum sodium concentration was 142 mEq/L, and now that she is in coma it is 118 mEq/L. Most likely she has been the victim of:

A. Air embolism.

B. Intracranial bleeding.

C. Renal loss of sodium.

D. Water loss.

E. Water retention.

167. A 72-year-old man with senile dementia falls at his nursing home and breaks his hip. He has an intertrochanteric fracture, which is treated by open reduction and internal fixation. He is placed on anticoagulants post-op. Five days after the procedure, he develops a massively distended colon. His abdomen is distended and tense, but not tender. His x-rays show the colon to be full of air, down to about the level of the sigmoid. After correction of his fluids and electrolytes, he needs:

A. Colonoscopy and long rectal tube.

B. Decompression by means of nasogastric suction.

C. Early ambulation to restore normal bowel motility.

D. Intravenous neostigmine.

E. Reversal of anticoagulation to allow urgent laparotomy.

168. A 17-year-old boy who is an insulin-dependent diabetic gets lost in the woods during a summer camp outing. He is found 3 days later in coma, with physical signs of dehydration and hyperventilation. The following laboratory report becomes available shortly after his workup begins in the emergency room of the nearest hospital: blood pH of 7.1, PCO_2 of 35, serum bicarbonate of 15, serum sodium 142, serum chloride 105. Those numbers tell you that he has:

   A. Laboratory evidence of loss of serum buffers.

   B. Metabolic acidosis with an anion gap.

   C. Metabolic acidosis with complete respiratory compensation.

   D. Primary metabolic alkalosis.

   E. Respiratory acidosis.

169. A 43-year-old man has a bloody bowel movement. He promptly reports to the ER, and while waiting to be seen he has another bloody evacuation. He reports the color of the blood in both of those as "dark red." A good look at his mouth and nose reveals no blood or lesions there, and the rest of a quick physical exam is equally noncontributory. A nasogastric tube is then inserted, and suction returns bloody gastric contents. The next step in the diagnostic workup should be:

   A. Arteriogram.

   B. Tagged red cell study.

   C. Technetium scan.

   D. Upper GI endoscopy.

   E. Upper GI series with barium.

170. A 67-year-old man comes to the office, with his wife, complaining of his inability to sleep. Pain in both calves keeps him awake. He finds some relief by dangling his feet, at which time his wife says his feet turn from very pale to deep purple. Asked about similar pain when he walks, they both point out that he knows he cannot walk more than a few yards without getting the same kind of pain. Physical exam shows shiny atrophic skin without hairs and no palpable pulses in his feet. The next step in the workup should be:

   A. Arteriogram.

   B. CT angio with spiral scan technology.

   C. Doppler studies, looking for a pressure gradient.

   D. Lipid profile.

   E. MRI angio.

171. A 39-year-old man with ascites, secondary to cirrhosis, develops diffuse abdominal pain. The problem began a couple of days ago, but the pain did not become significant until the third day. His physical examination is equivocal, with mild tenderness and perhaps a bit of rebound. He has mild fever and a minimal elevation in his WBC count. A sample of ascitic fluid sent for culture is reported to be growing a single organism. The next step in management should be:

   A. Antibiotics, guided by culture and sensitivities.

   B. Exploratory laparotomy.

   C. Ultrasound of the right upper quadrant.

   D. Serial CT scans of the abdomen.

   E. Vigorous use of diuretics until the ascites disappears.

172. A 34-year-old woman develops abdominal pain and shortly thereafter faints. When seen in the ER she has regained consciousness but is very weak, with profuse perspiration and a blood pressure of 85 over 50. Her hemoglobin is 8, and her abdomen is distended. There is no history of trauma. Thinking about the possibility of an ectopic pregnancy, she is asked about her GYN history. She is quite sure she is not pregnant, because she is on birth control pills, which she has faithfully taken since she was a teenager. This is a history suggestive of:

   A. Hepatic adenoma.

   B. Metastatic cancer to the liver.

   C. Primary hepatocellular carcinoma.

   D. Ruptured abdominal aortic aneurysm.

   E. Ruptured aneurysm of the hepatic artery.

173. A 79-year-old man reports fatigue and localized pain at specific places on several bones. X-rays show multiple, punched-out lytic lesions in the bones, and a complete blood count reveals that he is anemic. The next step in his diagnostic workup should be:

   A. Bence-Jones protein in urine, and serum immunoelectrophoresis.

   B. Bone marrow biopsies.

   C. MRI of the affected bones.

   D. Prostate-specific antigen (PSA).

   E. Radioisotope scan of the spleen.

174. A 17-year-old boy has a chest x-ray done because he fell and hurt his ribs. The radiologist reports that there are no rib fractures, but that the film shows "scalloping of the lower edge of the ribs." A subsequent physical exam shows significant hypertension, repeatedly measured on both arms. He has no palpable peripheral pulses in his legs. The next diagnostic study should be:

    A. Aldosterone and renin levels.

    B. Doppler studies of his renal vessels.

    C. Serum immunoelectrophoresis.

    D. Spiral CT scan enhanced with intravenous dye (CT angio).

    E. Twenty-four hour urinary collection for metanephrine levels.

175. A 3-year-old child is brought in by concerned parents because he has chronic constipation. He has no fecal soiling, and his abdomen is distended. When a rectal exam is done, there is explosive expulsion of stool and flatus, with relief of the abdominal distention. A barium enema shows a normal-looking distal colon, and a rather dilated proximal colon. The next diagnostic step should be:

    A. Colonoscopy.

    B. Comprehensive psychiatric evaluation.

    C. Full thickness biopsy of the rectal mucosa.

    D. Radioisotope scan of the lower abdomen.

    E. Sweat test.

176. A 12-year-old girl has a physical exam done prior to her acceptance at a summer camp. There is a faint heart murmur that triggers her referral to a pediatric cardiologist. The specialist instantly recognizes a faint pulmonary flow systolic murmur and a fixed split second heart sound. Upon direct questioning the family reports that indeed the girl has frequent colds and respiratory infections. You expect that an echocardiogram should show:

    A. Atrial septal defect.

    B. Classic ventricular septal defect up in the membranous portion.

    C. Diminished pulmonary vascular markings.

    D. Patent ductus arteriosus.

    E. Small ventricular septal defect near the apex.

177. Because of chronic cough and what might have been an episode of hemoptysis, a 45-year-old man has a chest x-ray taken. The radiologist reports a 3-cm coin lesion in the upper lobe of the right lung. The man has never smoked but has been exposed to secondhand smoke from his wife's long smoking habit. At one time he worked in a coal mine, and he has lived in an area where chronic fungal infections are common. The next step in management should be:

    A. Bronchoscopy and multiple biopsies.

    B. PET scan of the mediastinal nodes.

    C. Pulmonary function studies.

    D. Transthoracic needle biopsy.

    E. Try to locate an older chest x-ray to compare with this one.

178. A pediatric neurosurgeon takes a peek into his office waiting room and sees a child on hands and knees, holding his head lower than his torso. The child most likely has:

    A. Brain abscess.

    B. Chronic infection of the inner ear.

    C. Degenerative disease of the central nervous system.

    D. Ependymoma.

    E. Glioblastoma multiforme.

179. As the runners of a marathon approach the finish line, several bombs planted by terrorists explode at about knee level behind the spectators, creating dozens of traumatic lower extremity amputations. First responders should control bleeding by what method, and after initial hospital resuscitation, shock should be treated with what therapy?

    A. Direct pressure; whole blood.

    B. Direct pressure; packed red cells (RBCs).

    C. Tourniquets; whole fresh blood.

    D. Tourniquets; packed RBCs and fresh frozen plasma (FFP).

    E. Tourniquets; packed RBCs, FFP, and platelets in 1-1-1 ratio.

180. A patient with a history of episodes of severe paroxysmal hypertension is found on laboratory studies to be producing large amounts of epinephrine. Subsequent diagnostic imaging is expected to demonstrate that the source of that abnormality is located in the:

    A. Adrenal cortex.

    B. Adrenal medulla.

    C. Anterior pituitary gland.

    D. Paraspinal chromaffin tissue.

    E. Posterior pituitary gland.

Answer Key

Question number	Correct answer	Page/paragraph where explanation can be found
1.	(A)	3/1
2.	(A)	6/7
3.	(E)	6/6
4.	(E)	7/2
5.	(B)	8/2
6.	(D)	10/2
7.	(C)	10/6
8.	(C)	12/1
9.	(D)	13/4
10.	(C)	16/2
11.	(D)	17/8 and 18/1
12.	(E)	19/1
13.	(E)	20/3
14.	(C)	22/3
15.	(A)	29/1
16.	(D)	31/4
17.	(B)	13/3
18.	(A)	35/5
19.	(B)	37/4

Question number	Correct answer	Page/paragraph where explanation can be found
20.	(E)	39/5
21.	(D)	26/4
22.	(B)	43/5 and 44/1
23.	(E)	46/4 and 47/1
24.	(C)	48/7 and 49/1
25.	(D)	51/3
26.	(B)	54/4 and 51/1
27.	(D)	60/3
28.	(E)	63/1
29.	(C)	65/5 and 66/1
30.	(E)	69/3
31.	(B)	71/4
32.	(C)	74/4
33.	(A)	77/2
34.	(B)	81/3
35.	(C)	85/4
36.	(B)	86/5
37.	(A)	87/1
38.	(B)	90/1
39.	(B)	93/5
40.	(E)	97/2
41.	(E)	100/2 and 101/1
42.	(C)	105/1

Question number	Correct answer	Page/paragraph where explanation can be found
43.	(C)	107/4
44.	(E)	110/1
45.	(B)	113/3
46.	(A)	117/2
47.	(A)	119/2
48.	(E)	123/2
49.	(E)	124/6 and 125/1
50.	(A)	126/4
51.	(C)	107/6 and 108/1
52.	(C)	110/1 and 2
53.	(A)	113/4 and 114/1
54.	(B)	117/2
55.	(D)	119/1
56.	(A)	123/3
57.	(B)	125/2
58.	(C)	126/5 and 127/1
59.	(B)	130/2
60.	(B)	92/2
61.	(A)	134/2
62.	(C)	135/2
63.	(C)	137/6 and 138/1
64.	(E)	139/3
65.	(D)	141/3

Question number	Correct answer	Page/paragraph where explanation can be found
66.	(E)	147/4 and 148/1
67.	(A)	4/1
68.	(B)	6/2
69.	(D)	7/4
70.	(A)	9/4
71.	(E)	102/4
72.	(D)	14/2
73.	(C)	17/5 and 6
74.	(C)	102/5
75.	(B)	85/1 and 2
76.	(B)	19/5
77.	(C)	21/3
78.	(D)	24/2
79.	(C)	30/5
80.	(A)	33/1
81.	(A)	35/1
82.	(A)	36/4
83.	(D)	38/4
84.	(C)	40/4
85.	(C)	43/1
86.	(E)	46/3
87.	(D)	48/3
88.	(A)	50/3

Question number	Correct answer	Page/paragraph where explanation can be found
89.	(E)	54/1
90.	(A)	58/1
91.	(D)	64/4
92.	(C)	67/6
93.	(E)	70/3
94.	(D)	72/6
95.	(E)	76/4
96.	(D)	79/5
97.	(C)	66/4
98.	(C)	85/1 and 2
99.	(D)	87/3
100.	(B)	88/3
101.	(C)	92/4
102.	(D)	99/4
103.	(D)	102/2
104.	(C)	106/3
105.	(C)	88/2
106.	(E)	112/4
107.	(B)	118/2
108.	(D)	121/1
109.	(C)	124/6
110.	(D)	126/1
111.	(D)	127/3

Question number	Correct answer	Page/paragraph where explanation can be found
112.	(B)	132/2
113.	(A)	133/6 and 134/1
114.	(D)	137/1
115.	(A)	139/2
116.	(D)	140/4 and 141/1
117.	(C)	5/2 and 6/1
118.	(C)	6/6
119.	(B)	8/4 and 9/1
120.	(B)	10/4
121.	(B)	11/1
122.	(C)	12/3
123.	(C)	13/4
124.	(E)	16/3
125.	(C)	18/2
126.	(E)	19/1
127.	(D)	21/3 and 4
128.	(C)	23/3
129.	(D)	29/4 and 30/1
130.	(A)	32/2
131.	(D)	34/4
132.	(A)	35/6
133.	(C)	37/6
134.	(B)	39/7

Question number	Correct answer	Page/paragraph where explanation can be found
135.	(C)	41/6 and 42/1
136.	(D)	44/3
137.	(E)	45/3
138.	(C)	47/3
139.	(E)	49/2
140.	(E)	51/5
141.	(C)	57/1
142.	(B)	63/2
143.	(E)	66/3
144.	(C)	69/4
145.	(C)	72/3
146.	(B)	75/2
147.	(A)	77/4
148.	(B)	82/2
149.	(C)	86/1
150.	(C)	85/1 and 2, and 86/5
151.	(A)	50/3
152.	(E)	100/1
153.	(A)	131/2
154.	(A)	132/6
155.	(A)	132/4
156.	(C)	138/4
157.	(D)	22/2

Question number	Correct answer	Page/paragraph where explanation can be found
158.	(D)	73/2
159.	(A)	15/2
160.	(D)	102/2
161.	(B)	147/4 and 148/1
162.	(B)	138/5
163.	(D)	135/3 and 136/1
164.	(D)	43/4
165.	(B)	67/3
166.	(E)	57/2
167.	(A)	52/4
168.	(B)	60/1
169.	(D)	71/2
170.	(C)	112/6 and 113/1 and 2
171.	(A)	73/5
172.	(A)	76/3
173.	(A)	33/2
174.	(D)	94/2
175.	(C)	101/4
176.	(A)	105/4
177.	(E)	109/2
178.	(D)	133/5
179.	(E)	5/"Massive Bleeding" box
180.	(B)	91/3